HOUSE OF LORDS

S

AF765722

DMU 0428334 01 5

SELECT COMMITTEE ON
SCIENCE AND TECHNOLOGY

RESISTANCE TO ANTIBIOTICS

AND OTHER ANTIMICROBIAL AGENTS

REPORT

Ordered to be printed 17 March 1998

First Published 1998
Reprinted 1999
£13.30

HL Paper 81–I

DE MONTFORT UNIVERSITY LIBRARY

DE MONTFORT UNIVERSITY
LIBRARY
Acc. No 0428334015
Date 7-3-00
Loc./Form
Class 615.329
GRE

CONTENTS

References to evidence

Q refers to a question in oral evidence; p refers to a page of written evidence. All the evidence is printed in a separate volume, HL Paper 81–II, Session 1997–98.

SEVENTH REPORT

17 March 1998

By the Select Committee appointed to consider Science and Technology.

ORDERED TO REPORT

RESISTANCE TO ANTIBIOTICS
AND OTHER ANTIMICROBIAL AGENTS

CHAPTER 1 INTRODUCTION

1.1 Antibiotics have saved countless lives and transformed the practice of medicine since the first flowering of antimicrobial chemotherapy in the 1930s and '40s.[1] Many people are old enough to remember when these and other antimicrobial drugs were not available. Their memories include patients with pulmonary tuberculosis isolated in sanatoria until either they died or their disease healed itself; frequent postoperative wound infections; bone infections (osteomyelitis) followed by discharging sinuses requiring drainage for year after year; syphilis advancing to its late stages and ending in insanity despite the use of arsenical drugs; cases of tuberculous meningitis, invariably fatal; and simple cuts and scratches giving rise to fatal septicaemia.

1.2 L P Garrod wrote in 1968, "No one recently qualified, even with the liveliest imagination, can picture the ravages of bacterial infection which continued until little more than 30 years ago". Since then, many new antibacterial agents have been developed and antiviral chemotherapy, then in its infancy, has become possible for an increasing range of viral diseases. As well as its uses in the direct treatment of infection, antimicrobial chemotherapy has also helped to make possible medical advances such as transplantation and the treatment of many forms of cancer which carry a special risk of infection.

1.3 But the worm in the bud emerged early when, during the development of penicillin, the enzyme which destroys it was isolated and it was presciently predicted (by Abraham and Chain) that penicillin resistance would become a problem. So it has, and so also, at greatly varying intervals following its introduction, has resistance to each new antibiotic.

1.4 "Resistance" means that an organism ceases to be killed or inhibited by a drug. While antibiotics can cause, as can all active therapies, a wide range of adverse effects ranging from trivial to fatal, resistance is a special problem, since the agent loses its former efficacy and the future treatment of other patients is therefore jeopardised.[2] The problem of antibiotic resistance has now become a major concern in medicine throughout the world.

1.5 The fact of antibiotic resistance is widely known, though not so widely understood. In the United Kingdom, the aspect most talked about among the public at large is probably MRSA (methicillin-resistant *Staphylococcus aureus*), an infection associated principally with hospitals and nursing homes. Other aspects of the problem are familiar to the people affected: for instance, resistant TB (tuberculosis) is a major threat to people with AIDS, while resistant malaria is the scourge of Africa and the Far East. Both Houses of Parliament have debated MRSA and other

---

1 For terminology, see Box 1, and the glossary in Appendix 8.

2 Resistance should be distinguished from tolerance. When a patient develops tolerance to a drug, no other patient is affected; but a resistant organism can infect others.

Box 1

HISTORY AND TERMINOLOGY

Historically the concept of attacking invading organisms without harming the host was introduced at the turn of the century by the German Paul Ehrlich. This concept he called **chemotherapy**. The invading organisms he first studied were not bacteria but rather the protozoa that cause malaria and sleeping sickness; but in 1910 he made his great discovery of salvarsan (the 606th synthetic chemical he had tried) which was effective in treating the spirochaete (a type of bacterium) which causes syphilis. He called it a "magic bullet". In the 1930s the sulphonamide drugs were introduced: they were the first effective drugs that attacked the common bacteria such as streptococci and could cure pneumonia and meningitis, although they caused serious problems and side effects. They were not called antibiotics; they were known as "chemotherapeutic agents".

"**Antibiotic**" was the term originally applied to naturally occurring compounds such as penicillin which attacked infecting bacteria without harming the host. "Antibiotic" is now regularly used to refer to synthetic compounds as well as natural compounds, and to refer to antiviral as well as antibacterial drugs. In the public mind, however, "antibiotics" are still largely equated with penicillin.

Penicillin, the first antibiotic, was identified in a mould by Alexander Fleming in 1928; but it was not available for use until Florey and Chain and their colleagues purified it in 1940 and showed how effective it could be. Unlike the sulphonamides it seemed completely harmless to the host and very effective against many bacteria. As it was a naturally occurring product, not a synthetic chemical, it was not called a chemotherapeutic drug, although that would have been a perfectly correct description. It would also have been a correct general description to include not only all antibacterial agents but also agents against viruses, protozoa, worms and other parasites, with all of which our report is concerned. However, the word "chemotherapy" is now used and recognised by the public as the term to describe the drug treatment of cancer.

"Cancer chemotherapy" is a legitimate term if we regard cancerous cells as invasive, being therefore, like infecting organisms, foreign to the host. Cancer chemotherapy thus seeks to attack the invader without damaging the host. Chemotherapy against microbial infection is referred to as **antimicrobial chemotherapy**.

This report is concerned with various forms of antimicrobial chemotherapy, and mainly with antibacterial antibiotics, or **antibacterials**. It deals also with antiviral antibiotics, or **antivirals**; and with **antimalarial** and **anthelmintic** drugs.

For an historical account of the development of resistance to antibiotics, see the evidence of Professors Phillips and Roberts of the Royal College of Pathologists, p 453.

resistant infections in the past year or two (the Commons on 19 March 1997, the Lords on 4 November 1996). The Government are seized of the issue: it features in the Chief Medical Officer's annual reports for 1995 and 1996, and Ministers are awaiting advice on different aspects of it from the Standing Medical Advisory Committee and the Advisory Committee on the Microbiological Safety of Food (p 373). So we bring the matter before the House confident that it deserves Parliamentary time and attention. This enquiry has been an alarming experience, which leaves us convinced that resistance to antibiotics and other anti-infective agents constitutes a major threat to public health, and ought to be recognised as such more widely than it is at present.

1.6 We begin our report with a brief account of what resistance is and why it matters; for more on these questions, we refer the reader to a recent report by the Parliamentary Office of Science and Technology, *Diseases Fighting Back* (October 1994). We consider how far resistance can be controlled, and how. We then proceed to consider the evidence we have received on the various means of control: prudent use of antimicrobial agents in human medicine (Chapter 2) and in animals (Chapter 3); infection control (Chapter 4) and disease surveillance (Chapter 5); and development of new drugs (Chapter 6) and vaccines (Chapter 7). Chapter 8 considers the special problems of resistance in viruses, and Chapter 9 considers international issues including malaria. Chapter 10 considers the sources of support for research and data-collection. Our recommendations are set out in Chapter 11, and summarised in Chapter 12. Appendix 7 contains notes on some important antimicrobial agents, Appendix 8 a glossary of other terms, and Appendix 9 a list of acronyms.

What is resistance?

1.7 All antibiotic resistance has a genetic basis. Some organisms are inherently resistant to many antibiotics ("innate resistance"). This resistance probably evolved as a response to exposure to antibiotics present in the natural environment. Many such organisms pose no threat to healthy people, but may become important pathogens in vulnerable patients in hospital. Examples include the Pseudomonas species and some Enterococci.

1.8 Acquired resistance can arise by a number of diverse mechanisms:

(i) Mutational resistance. These mutations have occurred randomly in a small proportion of the particular bacterial population. The most familiar example is seen in the bacterium causing tuberculosis, where a few organisms are naturally resistant to, for example, streptomycin. In the presence of streptomycin as a single antibiotic these resistant organisms soon become the dominant population.

(ii) By horizontal transfer of genes determining resistance from one organism to another. This can occur by the direct transfer (conjugation) between bacteria of genetic material carried on small pieces of DNA (plasmids) situated within the bacterial cell but outside the bacterial chromosome, or by similar pieces of DNA carried on a bacterial virus, a bacteriophage (transduction), or by direct transfer of naked DNA (transformation).

1.9 While these mechanisms have been known for many years, what has emerged more recently is knowledge of the great frequency and flexibility with which bacteria are able to exchange genetic material. and the crucial importance of these mechanisms in bacterial evolution. It is now known, for example, that genetic interchange can take place between a much more diverse variety of organisms than was formerly thought. and is probably a common event in the natural world. There is a global pool of resistance genes which can spread between different bacterial populations occupying different habitats, e.g. between man, animals and the environment. Genes carrying antibiotic resistance factors are easily able to spread if the host organism gains an evolutionary advantage in acquiring them. The importance of these processes for antibiotic resistance in man and animals is that, by whichever process genes for resistance have been acquired, the presence of an antibiotic in the environment of the bacterium imposes "selection pressure" and encourages resistance to spread. The antibiotic kills all susceptible bacteria, thereby "selecting out" the resistant strain; in this way a previously minor population of antibiotic-resistant organisms rapidly becomes dominant. Although there are enormous variations in the speed with which resistance to any antibiotic emerges, and in its geographical spread once it has emerged, it is indisputable that resistance has developed to many new agents after their introduction, with consequent diminution or actual loss of their former value to medicine. Thus has appeared the vicious circle repeatedly witnessed during the last half century, in which the value of each new antibiotic has been progressively eroded by resistance, leading to the introduction of a new and usually more expensive agent, only for this in its turn to suffer the same fate.

Clinical resistance

1.10 Bacterial species differ greatly in their inherent susceptibility or resistance to various antibiotics. There is also a range of susceptibility within any species, so that some organisms are more susceptible than others. Clinical resistance, i.e. whether the antibiotic will or will not work in a patient or animal, is a more complex concept in which many other factors are involved such as the precise location of the infection, the distribution of the drug in body fluids and the state of the patient's immune system.

1.11 Resistance is measured in the clinical microbiology laboratory by qualitative or quantitative methods which attempt to relate the test results to the expected effect in clinical practice, taking into account such factors as the range of serum concentrations achieved when the antibiotic is administered. Most laboratories use an agar disc susceptibility test in which isolates (i.e. samples) are categorised as susceptible, resistant or intermediate.

1.12 There is much continued discussion about the best methods of antibiotic testing, about quality control and about international agreement on methods. In practice, the results of these pragmatic tests often relate well to clinical success or failure, for example in tuberculosis and in gonorrhoea.

1.13 At a more basic level, the biochemical mechanisms responsible for antibiotic resistance have been analysed in great detail. Resistance arises (i) if the bacteria can inactivate the drug before it reaches its target within the bacterial cell; (ii) if the outer layers of the cell are impermeable, and prevent the drug from entering; (iii) if the drug enters but is then pumped back out again ("efflux"); (iv) if the target is altered so that it is no longer recognised by the antibiotic, or (v) if the bacteria acquire an alternative metabolic pathway that renders the antibiotic's target redundant ("by-pass"). Although some hundreds of resistances are known, virtually all can be ascribed to one of these five broad types of mechanism. See Figure 1, which represents the antibiotic as a bullet and the target as a roundel.[3]

Cross-infection

1.14 Bacteria inhabit a global environmental pool in which resistant bacteria, and genes transferring antibiotic resistance between bacteria, can and do spread easily between people and animals. A continuous process of exchange of genes takes place within the microbial world. The two variable factors affecting the spread of antibiotic resistance are the selection pressure exerted by antibiotic use, and the ease with which resistant organisms are able to spread between people by "cross-infection".

The international dimension

1.15 Because the amount of interaction between human populations, and with them their commensal[4] microbes, varies greatly, the type and frequency of antibiotic resistance in any particular organism differs greatly between geographical locations. In the longer term, however, once antibiotic resistance is established in an organism, it spreads with lesser or greater speed throughout the world. Modern methods of molecular epidemiology have enabled the spread of bacteria to be tracked and it is clear that bacteria, some of them carrying antibiotic resistance factors, can spread between countries and continents with phenomenal speed in this era of mass travel.

---

[3] We are indebted for this simple account of a complex matter, and for the Figure, to Dr David Livermore, Head of the PHLS Antibiotic Reference Unit. See also *Diseases Fighting Back*, Parliamentary Office of Science and Technology, October 1994; and the memoranda of the Association of Medical Microbiologists (p 2) and the Society for General Microbiology (p 485).

[4] Commensal microbes, or "flora", are the numerous and diverse micro-organisms which inhabit the skin, nose, mouth and gut. They do not normally cause disease in healthy people.

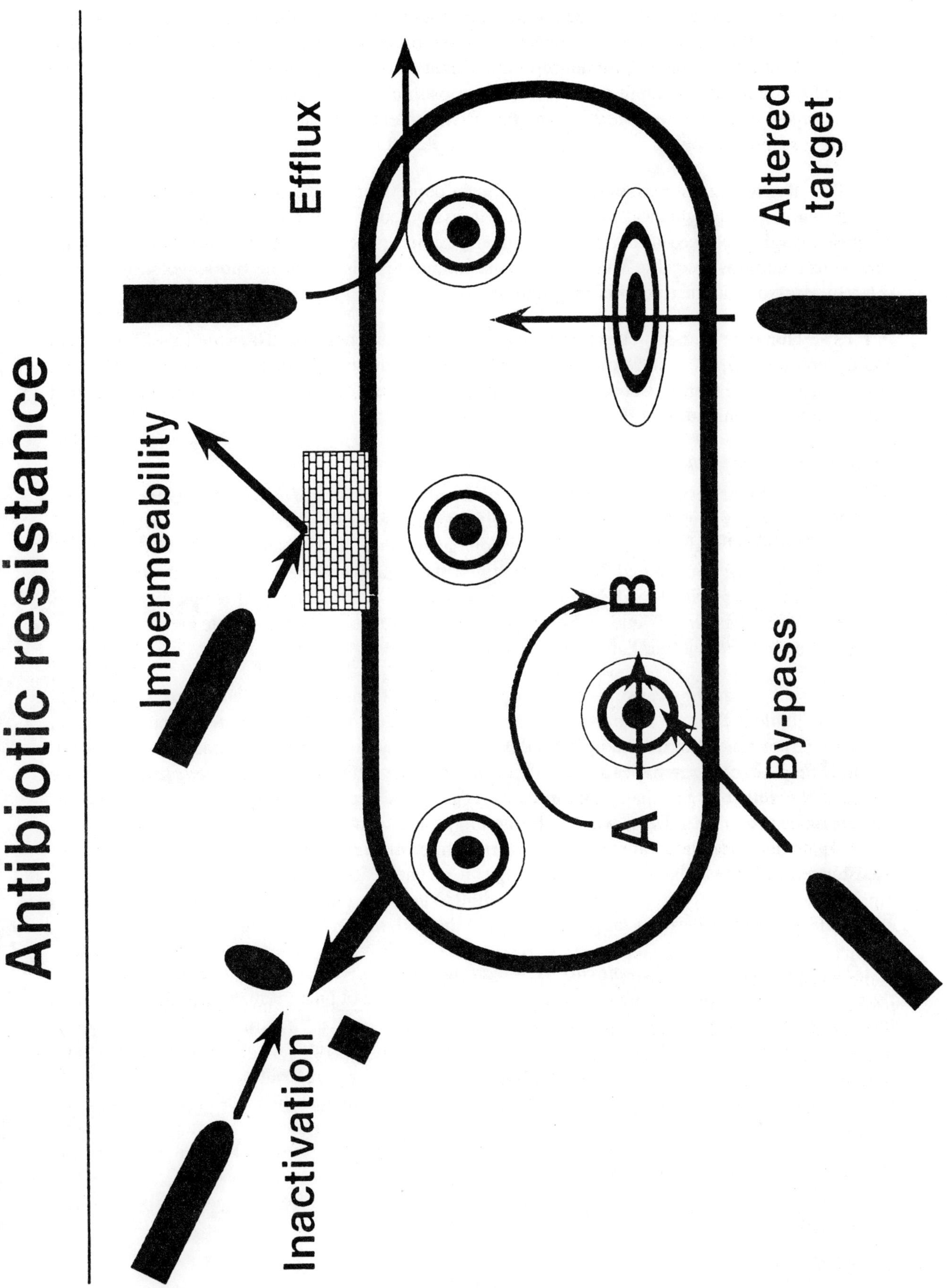
Antibiotic resistance
Impermeability
Efflux
Altered target
By-pass
A
B
Inactivation

Hospital infection

1.16 Although antibiotic resistance is encountered everywhere, there are special problems in hospitals and other health care institutions. Many organisms which are part of the normal commensal flora of the body pose an important threat to patients whose resistance is lowered by reason of illness, surgery, administration of immunosuppressant drugs, or extremes of age. Many of these organisms, such as VRE (vancomycin-resistant enterococcus[5]), are highly resistant, and even previously susceptible species can easily be replaced by resistant strains.

1.17 The hospital environment, especially in departments such as intensive care units and neonatal units, operates as an epidemiological pressure cooker for the emergence of resistance, combining high infective risks in immunologically compromised patients who are also undergoing invasive procedures, frequent spread of infection, and high usage of antibiotics exerting strong selective pressure on the microbial population.

1.18 Some organisms causing hospital infection, such as MRSA (methicillin-resistant *Staphylococcus aureus*—see below), may also become a significant problem outside hospitals; and, even if they do not, their presence in the normal flora of people in the community is an important factor in the dissemination of these resistant strains.

Does antibiotic resistance matter?

1.19 Antibiotic resistance threatens mankind with the prospect of a return to the pre-antibiotic era. This will not, of course, happen overnight. It is a relatively slow but inexorable process, patchy in its effects but already under way. The options available for the treatment of infections have everywhere become constrained. In some locations, the organisms causing several life-threatening infections are now resistant to all available antibiotics, so that for patients suffering these illnesses the antibiotic era has already ended. Some examples will serve to emphasise the great importance of resistance in bacterial, viral and parasitic disease.

1.20 The organisms causing gut infections such as **typhoid and bacillary dysentery** are peculiarly liable to become antibiotic resistant. These organisms also acquire resistance to several antibiotics (multiple drug resistance, MDR) with great facility, so that Salmonella species, for example, can become resistant to 8 or 10 antibiotics. The genes conferring these properties are transferred together as a package, and infections caused by these strains are untreatable by any of the antibiotics involved. Thus, when it became possible to treat typhoid fever with antibiotics, chloramphenicol and later amoxycillin or trimethoprim were widely and successfully used. Resistance to all these agents emerged so that in recent years it has been necessary to employ ciprofloxacin as the only effective agent remaining to us. Now ciprofloxacin-resistant typhoid has emerged in many places and is at present causing an epidemic in Tajikistan.

1.21 **Pneumococcus (*Streptococcus pneumoniae*)** is a universal organism often carried in the nose and throat of healthy people. It is the most common cause of pneumonia in adults and children throughout the world, a major cause of otitis media, and one of the three most common causes of bacterial meningitis. Pneumococcal meningitis is an especially serious form, with a high mortality and a high probability of deafness and other neurological consequences in its survivors. For nearly 40 years after penicillin was introduced, the pneumococcus remained fully susceptible. Resistance then emerged and is now in the process of disseminating throughout the world.[6] In some countries resistant strains are already dominant; in the United Kingdom at present they are an increasing problem. A few penicillin-resistant pneumococci are highly resistant and these strains often show multiple resistance to other antibiotics. Few options are available for treating meningitis caused by

---

[5] See the evidence of Dr H F Kennedy and Dr J R Michie of the Royal Hospital for Sick Children, Glasgow (p 549).

[6] See the evidence of Professor Keith Klugman, Director of the South African Institute for Medical Research (p 426).

such strains, and the agents remaining are unavailable in many poorer countries, so that pneumococcal meningitis has become effectively untreatable in these places.

1.22 The lives of patients with **meningococcal meningitis** were first saved by sulphonamides in the late 1930s. By the 1970s too many strains were sulphonamide-resistant for these drugs to remain in use for a life-threatening infection and penicillin became universally, and effectively, the treatment of choice. Penicillin resistance in meningococci has now emerged in a few places. Its presence anywhere is serious; spread to the meningitis belt of Africa (a wide geographical area subject to large epidemics every few years) would constitute a major disaster in world health.

1.23 Staphylococci are omnipresent on our skins; they are normally benign but capable of causing infections ranging from a boil to life-threatening septicaemia. **Methicillin-resistant *Staphylococcus aureus* (MRSA)**, often also resistant to many other antibiotics, has become highly prevalent in many hospitals and nursing homes.[7] Only vancomycin and related drugs, toxic, expensive and not always effective agents, remain for their treatment; and the first isolates of vancomycin-resistant *S. aureus*[8] (VRSA) have already been reported in Japan and the USA.

1.24 **Gonorrhoea** provides one of the clearest examples of the successive loss of one antibiotic after another because of the inexorable advance of antibiotic resistance. At first sulphonamides were successful but resistance rapidly emerged. A form of penicillin resistance which could be overcome by increasing the dose followed, with a progressive increase in the amount of penicillin needed to effect a cure. Later still, gonococci acquired the ability to make penicillinase, completely vitiating the effect of penicillin in gonococcal infection caused by these strains. Many other formerly effective agents have suffered the same fate, leading to the need for progressive changes in national and WHO recommendations for the treatment of this common worldwide infection. Many of the changes have involved increasingly expensive drugs.

1.25 **Tuberculosis** (TB) kills around three million people each year, more than any other infectious disease. Resistance to the first antibiotics effective against tuberculosis was detected as soon as they were introduced. How this could be prevented, by using two or three agents in combination, was then rapidly discovered, and a series of meticulous trials by the United Kingdom Medical Research Council established regimens of treatment which were highly successful both in curing patients and in preventing the emergence of resistance. Resistance has remained rare in countries such as the United Kingdom, where these regimens are generally followed under a well-established system for diagnosis and treatment. Sadly, however, resistance has become important in many countries because, for many reasons, the established regimens have often been neglected by doctors and by patients.

1.26 Multi-drug resistant (MDR) tuberculosis is a newer and different problem, found especially but not exclusively in patients with HIV infection, carrying a high mortality and extremely difficult to treat. Here is another example, in which our antibiotic options are nearly exhausted and when tuberculosis again becomes "the captain of all these men of death".[9] MDR tuberculosis is at present rare in the United Kingdom.[10]

1.27 **Malaria** is thought to cause two million deaths and several hundred million new infections annually throughout the world. A variety of resistance patterns has emerged, creating serious constraints on the options available for both treatment and prevention. In highly endemic areas it is becoming increasingly difficult to treat life-threatening disease in children. Most

---

7 See the evidence of Dr R Hill of King's College Hospital, p 417.

8 These isolates have also been characterised as "vancomycin-intermediate" (VISA), because, although their susceptibility is reduced, they are not absolutely resistant. We were told in the USA that these isolates, though alarming in their own right, were not what VRSA had been expected to look like.

9 John Bunyan, *The Life and Death of Mr Badman*.

10 Dr B Bannister at Coppetts Wood Hospital sees 50 new cases of TB each year; of these, two or three are MDR–TB, usually in people from Turkey or central Africa (p 377). Professor D A Mitchison of St George's Hospital puts the total number of cases of MDR–TB in the United Kingdom at present at fewer than 20 (p 432).

important is chloroquine resistance, now widespread in many continents. Chloroquine resistance has necessitated a return to the oldest of all chemotherapeutic agents, quinine, but multiple resistance, including partial resistance to quinine, is now a major problem in SE Asia. The consequences of the current degree of malarial resistance are massive, especially in Africa where Ministries of Health have annual budgets of a few dollars per head. See Chapter 9 below.

1.28 **Viruses** can also become resistant to the drugs used in their treatment. This takes place inside the cells of the patient, within which the virus multiplies. Viruses such as HIV replicate very rapidly and minor variations of the genome occur with each multiplication, leading to a genetically heterogeneous population of viral particles. It is inevitable that, in the presence of an antiviral drug, variants with increased resistance to its action will show a selective advantage and will soon become the majority species. Much effort is now being undertaken to find how best to use antiviral drugs in ways which make it more difficult for resistance to emerge. See Chapter 8 below.

1.29 The impact of antibiotic resistance on our ability to treat some important infections is summarised in Box 2.

1.30 There are some exceptions to the general onward march of resistance. For example, *Streptococcus pyogenes* (group A haemolytic streptococcus) has so far remained susceptible to penicillin, although it is often resistant to several other agents. Likewise, resistance has rarely been reported among the chlamydia, an important cause of genital and eye infections including trachoma; and the causative organism of syphilis (*Treponema pallidum*) has remained susceptible to penicillin. We do not attempt to describe the problem of resistance as it affects all pathogens, but have concentrated on those of particular importance for world health.

Can resistance be controlled?

1.31 How to tackle the problems of resistance depends critically on the answer to a question on which science is divided: can the rise in the proportion of resistant strains be reversed, or at least slowed down, or is it inexorable?

1.32 Professor David Reeves, President of the Association of Medical Microbiologists (AMM), is an optimist. "There is plenty of evidence that, if you remove the selection pressure, the organisms will slowly revert [to susceptibility], some types of organisms more quickly than others and to certain antibiotics more quickly than to others" (Q 23, cp McGavock Q 675). Dr Peter Davey, Reader in Clinical Pharmacology at Ninewells Hospital, Dundee, gave us a table of supporting evidence for the proposition that resistance is dependent on usage (p 145), but produced at least one potential confounding variable for each point. Professor A Percival, Professor of Clinical Bacteriology at Liverpool University, put it starkly: "The concept that antibiotic resistance is related somehow to the amount of use is critical, because, if it is not true, then we have no chance of controlling it...Although everybody believes that, the evidence to support it and to demonstrate it in a scientifically acceptable way is largely lacking...worldwide" (Q 73).

1.33 In marked contrast with Professor Reeves' optimism was the approach of Dr Bruce Levin, a population biologist from Emory University, whom we met in Atlanta. He believes that resistance is a one-way street: even if antibiotic use is cut back sharply, the proportion of resistant strains wanes slowly if at all; even moderate use still imposes heavy selective pressure; and, if use is resumed, resistance rises again more rapidly than before. As he put it, "We are committed to an arms race"; disarmament is not an option. See Appendix 6.

1.34 Countries with firmer controls on the supply and use of antibiotics, and more rigorous infection control, have lower rates of resistant strains, and it is generally assumed that these things are connected. "Holland and Denmark have amongst the lowest incidence of MRSA, due to their effective antibiotic and infection control policies" (PHLS p 42). "Spain has the highest consumption of anti-infectives *per capita* in Europe, and one of the worst records of antibiotic resistance" (ABPI p 176).

Box 2

EXAMPLES OF VALUABLE ANTIBIOTIC THERAPIES NOW LOST OR IMPERILLED BY THE SPREAD OF RESISTANCE

Organism	**Disease**	**Agents lost or threatened**[11]
Pneumococcus	Pneumonia, otitis, meningitis	Penicillin; many others
Meningococcus	Meningitis, septicaemia	Sulphonamides; (penicillin)
Haemophilus influenzae	Meningitis	Ampicillin, chloramphenicol
Staphylococcus aureus	Wound infection, sepsis	Penicillin, penicillinase-resistant penicillins, others
Salmonella typhi	Typhoid fever	Most relevant agents
Shigella spp.	Bacillary dysentery	Most relevant agents
Gonococcus	Gonorrhoea	Sulphonamides, penicillin, tetracycline; (ciprofloxacin)
Plasmodium falciparum	Severe malaria	Chloroquine, pyrimethamine; (mefloquine, quinine)
E. coli (coliforms)	Urinary infection, septicaemia	Ampicillin, trimethoprim, others

1.35 Slowing the take-over of resistant strains is one thing; eradicating them once they have arrived is another, and seems to be easier for some organisms than for others. Resistance in the gonococcus to penicillin (PHLS p 68), and in *Strep. pyogenes* to erythromycin (AMM p 9, Finch p 187), can be reduced; resistance in *Staph. aureus* to methicillin (PHLS p 43) and in *E. coli* to streptomycin (PHLS p 52), once prevalent, appears to be stable.

1.36 Throughout our enquiry we have listened for stories of success in reversing the rise in the proportion of resistant strains. Only two such stories have been rigorously researched and written up (Anderson Q 687). In Finland, an increase in resistance of Group A streptococci to erythromycin around 1990 was countered by a policy restricting the use of macrolides in favour of alternative drugs. Consumption was reduced by nearly a half by 1992, and the rate of resistance was nearly halved by 1996. Dr Davey told a similar tale from Iceland (Q 261), where a problem with penicillin-resistant pneumococci was associated with day-care centres for children. "There was an information campaign aimed at the public and doctors, saying that giving antibiotics to children too frequently at day-care centres was not a good idea. They did reduce the antibiotic prescribing, and they have reduced the transmission of these resistant bugs".

1.37 According to the Department of Health, "The role of the use of antimicrobials in the development of antimicrobial resistance is undoubted. Those countries with high usage and uncontrolled availability of 'over the counter' antibiotics tend to have higher levels of antimicrobial resistance, whereas Denmark for instance has seen a dramatic reduction in the prevalence of antibiotic resistant micro-organisms since tight controls on antimicrobial usage, together with strict infection control procedures, were introduced" (p 342).[12] On the basis of the Danish experience, the Chief Medical Officer considers that it should be an objective of Government strategy "to reduce the prevalence of micro-organisms resistant to current drugs" (Q 756).

---

11 Because of the widely variable distribution of antibiotic resistance at any time, a clear distinction between 'lost' and 'threatened' cannot be made. An antibiotic now useless in one place may still be valuable in another. Resistance to the agents in parentheses is so far uncommon.

12 Dr Rosamund Williams of WHO (Q 132) told us that the Danish strategy included surveillance of resistance and usage, strict national prescribing guidelines with follow-up of doctors who infringe them, and isolation and screening of infected persons. The Minister for Public Health said that the Department of Health are "very interested" in the Danish approach (Q 755).

1.38 As for malaria, Dr David Warhurst of the London School of Hygiene and Tropical Medicine told us, "There is evidence that, if drugs are not used, some of these [resistant malarial] organisms will probably get back to their pre-existing state" (Q 493). Dr Deenan Pillay, Director of the PHLS Antiviral Susceptibility Reference Laboratory in Birmingham, told a similar tale from virology (Q 614).

1.39 So what is the policy-maker to conclude? We suggest that the following propositions conform with the present state of knowledge:

(i) Any antimicrobial agent must be expected to encounter resistance sooner or later.

(ii) Resistant strains will take longer to emerge and spread if antimicrobial use is controlled and prudent from the start.

(iii) Improving the control of antimicrobial use can be expected to slow down the rise in the proportion of resistant strains. In the case of certain pathogens (e.g. streptococci, pneumococci, gonococci), the proportion may even fall; but this must not be expected to happen in every case. If, following an improvement in control and a fall in resistance, control is once again relaxed, reversion to high levels of resistance may be swift.

1.40 Why reducing the selective pressure of antimicrobials sometimes brings down the level of resistance and sometimes does not, scientists cannot yet say with certainty. As noted above, in cases where it does, it may be because resistance, though in itself an advantage from the microbe's point of view, confers a collateral burden such that, in the absence of selective pressure, the resistant strain is at an evolutionary disadvantage (i.e. in terms of "survival of the fittest", the resistant strain is less fit), and susceptible strains take over again. Where resistance does not evolve away, it may be because the resistant strain has undergone a secondary adaptation and evolved around the burden, so that in the absence of selective pressure it is no longer at a disadvantage. Alternatively, it may be because the plasmid carrying the gene which confers the resistance in question also carries, as a package, genes which code for resistance to other agents (e.g. Salmonella may carry packages of resistance to as many as 10 antibiotics); if just one of these agents remains in use, selective pressure will keep all the resistances in the package at high levels.

1.41 These rules of thumb, though rough and ready, are based on evidence from leaders in the field in both the United Kingdom and the USA; and those with whom we have spoken readily admit that knowledge in this area is incomplete and somewhat anecdotal. The case for continued research is clear: see Chapter 10 below.

Acknowledgements

1.42 The enquiry which led to this report was conducted between July 1997 and March 1998 by Sub-Committee I, whose members are listed in Appendix 1. They received evidence from the organisations and individuals listed in Appendix 2, to all of whom we are grateful for their time and trouble. They paid two visits to the Headquarters of the Public Health Laboratory Service (PHLS) in Colindale, where Professor Brian Duerden, Deputy Director, and numerous members of PHLS staff, were extremely helpful: see Appendices 3 and 4. They visited King's College Hospital, on Denmark Hill; we are grateful to Professor Mark Casewell, then Professor of Medical Microbiology, and to members of the medical and nursing staff, for organising a very informative visit: see Appendix 5. In November, four members visited the USA: Appendix 6 describes the visit, and acknowledges the numerous people who gave generously of their time to make it worthwhile. We acknowledge the help of Sub-Committee I's Specialist Advisers, Professor Harold Lambert, Emeritus Professor of Microbial Diseases at St George's Hospital, Tooting, and Professor Richard Wise, Professor of Clinical Microbiology at Birmingham City Hospital. Finally, we are grateful to the Parliamentary Office of Science and Technology (POST), for the report *Diseases Fighting Back* noted above, and for a report on *Vaccines and their Future Role in Public Health.*

CHAPTER 2 PRUDENT USE IN HUMAN MEDICINE

2.1 The evidence set out above suggests that one way to tackle drug resistance in the short term is to work towards appropriate and prudent usage of the drugs themselves. In the longer term there may be new drugs and vaccines (see Chapters 6 and 7); but every doctor, dentist and veterinary surgeon can, it seems, affect the situation for better or worse from day to day by more or less appropriate prescribing.[13]

2.2 It must be recognised at once that, even without the issue of resistance, use of medicines is a three-cornered battlefield. Doctors want the freedom to do the best for their patients; those who pay for health care, whether governments or insurers or the patients themselves, want good care at low cost; and pharmaceutical manufacturers want to maximise the return to their shareholders. Discussion of the impact of usage on resistance cannot be divorced from this context.

Present use in the United Kingdom

2.3 In the United Kingdom, most antimicrobials used in human medicine are prescribed by GPs (general practitioners, or family doctors). The Association of Medical Microbiologists (AMM - QQ 45–52, p 9) told us that in England alone, GPs prescribe 270m defined daily doses each year—"enough antibiotics to treat every man, woman and child in England for five days a year". This is much more than is administered in hospitals (though data do not permit a precise comparison, and even if they did one would not be comparing like with like). This figure is derived from Prescription Pricing Authority (PPA) data for 1992–94; the same data show an annual increase in prescribing of 5 per cent over the previous three years, with no simultaneous increase in infectious disease to explain it. They also show a tendency to prescribe newer drugs instead of older ones. However the AMM believe around 80 per cent of antimicrobial prescribing in United Kingdom general practice to be "fully justified" (Q 45).

2.4 The Association of the British Pharmaceutical Industry (ABPI) gave us a different set of figures. In 1996, United Kingdom GPs wrote 51m antibiotic prescriptions, which, though a lot, was 2.5m fewer than the previous year. They conclude, "The message about not prescribing antibiotics in diseases that are probably viral appears to be getting through" (p 177).

2.5 The Department of Health produce yet more figures, and analyse them in detail (p 343). Between 1991 and 1996 in England, the number of prescription items for antibacterials increased by only 7 per cent, and the net ingredient cost by only 4 per cent, both much less than the figures for all drugs; between 1995 and 1996 both figures went down, as noted by the ABPI. However there were wide variations from drug to drug. The group which gives "most cause for concern" is the fluoroquinolones: over the five years, use rose by 48 per cent, and cost by 81 per cent. "Ciprofloxacin is the market leader in a group of drugs which is heavily promoted". Use of penicillins rose by 13 per cent; the Department find this "disappointing", though they suggest possible innocent explanations.[14] Use of macrolides rose only marginally, but their cost rose by 58 per cent, probably because erythromycin, the original macrolide, lost market share to newer and more expensive macrolides with additional applications (e.g. azithromycin). "The newer macrolides are heavily promoted". The Department produce further figures to show that antibiotic prescribing varies widely between health authorities.

2.6 From his experience in Oxfordshire, Dr Richard Mayon-White, a Consultant in Communicable Disease Control, considers the antibiotic prescribing of United Kingdom GPs to be "conservative" (p 110). However local monitoring has revealed "wide variations" in prescribing of expensive drugs such as ciprofloxacin. Dr Hugh McGavock, Director of the Drug Utilisation Research Unit at The Queen's University of Belfast, detects a bell-curve (Q 660): "some doctors

---

13 What we have to say about doctors should be taken to apply *mutatis mutandis* to dentists. Veterinary practice is discussed separately in the next chapter.

14 Demographic factors, or an increase in repeat treatments due to rising resistance.

accepting the guidelines perfectly, the majority moderately well, and some doctors on the far side of the curve hardly paying any attention to them". The Royal College of General Practitioners (RCGP) stand by their profession: "Given the context of diagnostic uncertainty, current prescribing practice of GPs is in general more beneficial than harmful in the care of individual patients" (p 166). However, "There is sufficient evidence of widespread variation in the utilisation of antibiotics to suggest that there is scope for further reduction of their use by some practitioners". Dr Davey is more sceptical about GP prescribing. "We have intense debates about whether children with otitis media should receive antibiotics, or people with sore throats. But our work would suggest that the majority of patients to receive antibiotics...just have runny noses, where there is no evidence that they benefit" (Q 265).

2.7 There is no equivalent to PPA data for hospitals (DH p 342); all one can say for certain is that hospitals dispense a much smaller volume of antimicrobials than are prescribed in general practice. According to the Department of Health, 15–20 per cent of hospital expenditure on drugs goes on antimicrobials; and around one in-patient in four receives at least one course of antibiotics. The AMM produced, by different routes, two different "ballpark" figures: on the one hand, 1–2m daily doses per year in English hospitals, or on the other the significantly higher figure of something under 5m in the whole United Kingdom (p 9). 20–30 per cent of hospital usage of antimicrobials is for prophylaxis against infection during surgery; and, according to the AMM, "courses given are often longer than necessary". Dr Davey also has doubts about current practice in this area (p 152; QQ 267, 272): "At the moment I do not think we have sufficient debate about what level of benefit [in terms of reduced risk from infection] justifies the use of antibiotics".[15]

Towards more prudent use

2.8 The AMM believe that, by a significant and sustained campaign of education, it might be possible to eliminate the "small proportion" of United Kingdom GP prescribing which they believe to be completely unjustified, and to reduce the larger proportion which "is perhaps not founded on the best evidence-based practice but may be justified by medical, cultural or psychological reason". They warned us, "The continuing legitimate use of antibiotics in humans may still sustain and might even increase the amount of resistance"[16]; to say nothing of resistance continuing to be generated in animals, and in humans in other countries where imprudent use persists. However, "the medical profession must put its own house in order before it can expect others to do so" (pp 8–13). On the other hand Dr Davey, who believes that more than half of GP prescribing is justified by nothing more than a runny nose, would happily "let the people with the sore throats get antibiotics but concentrate on the people who do not have any clinical signs which warrant antibiotics" (Q 265).

2.9 These contrasting positions present the question, What constitutes prudence? The RCGP insist that, although doctors have a national, strategic responsibility for public health, this cannot override their primary responsibility to the individual patient (p 167, Q 280). Dr Davey put it more bluntly: "I would much rather...some people received unnecessary treatment than we end up with somebody dying" (Q 268). Dr McGavock was equally blunt on the other side of the dilemma: "[Over-prescription] is a situation that really must be changed if we wish to preserve the antimicrobial era...it may well go on, but if it does our grandchildren will curse us for wasting this limited human resource" (Q 647). Witnesses have pointed to various ways to resolve this dilemma; we consider them below.

---

15 Cp BMA: "Antibiotic misuse is common and studies have suggested that up to 70 per cent of treatment courses are unnecessary or inappropriate. Therapy is often unnecessarily prolonged and prophylaxis is often inappropriate or given at the wrong time" (p 381). The National Committee for Microbiology also express concern in this area (p 541).

16 Cp Glaxo Wellcome: "The recent lessons learnt from anti-retroviral chemotherapy have demonstrated the very powerful effects that natural selection can have, even when prescribing is entirely appropriate and patients are highly motivated to comply with treatment" (p 407).

Formularies, policies and guidelines

2.10 A formulary is a list of available drugs, or of drugs recommended from among those available; a policy gives guidance or instruction on when and how they are to be used. In the United Kingdom, most hospitals and some general practices have at least a formulary of antibacterials recommended for local use, and some hospitals have antibacterial policies.

2.11 The PHLS presented us with the findings of a survey of clinical audit in hospitals in England and Wales, in the context of MRSA (p 41). They found that formularies vary widely in form and content, and "are drawn up with little involvement of the junior staff; comments are often not invited"; that communication of antibiotic policies to new staff is often poor; and that audit of prescribing is often irregular, infrequent and unstructured. The AMM recommend that all hospitals and general practices should have both formularies and policies. These should be produced in a way which gives the doctor "ownership"; and they should be supported by strong encouragement from the health departments, and by audit.

2.12 Policies may operate at any level, from local to global (RCGP p 167; DH p 344; Petrie Q 669). They may reflect the threat of resistance by recommending rotation or combination of drugs (Davey Q 263, Spencer p 519, Tyrell p 528), or by avoiding certain drugs altogether (PHLS p 52). They may be supported by restrictive reporting,[17] by financial incentives (recommended by Dr McGavock, Q 658) and even by compulsion (resisted by Professor Petrie, Q 674). They may be more or less flexible; Glaxo Wellcome advocate flexibility, "to enable nimble local responses to changes in resistance patterns" (p 407). Box 3 gives examples of good practice in this area which have come to our notice.

2.13 A policy is not a panacea. It must be sound in itself, and must be implemented conscientiously and intelligently. It must also be policed: see below, paragraph 2.34. Dr R C Spencer, of the Public Health Laboratory at Bristol Royal Infirmary, points out that policies depend on surveillance, to indicate what the infecting organism is most likely to be, and what resistances it is likely to exhibit (p 513). We consider surveillance in Chapter 5. As for implementation, Professor Percival gave us the example of a policy drawn up for severe community-acquired pneumonia; it was applied to pneumonia of all kinds, and is now blamed for "a tremendous increase in *Clostridium difficile* side-effects" (Q 104).

2.14 The pharmaceutical industry strongly prefer evidence-based guidelines for appropriate prescribing, rather than crude injunctions to prescribe less. In some situations, they say, certain drugs should be withdrawn, in others they should be used in combination (particularly for TB and HIV) or rotated; in others new and better agents should be used. Guidelines must be based on evidence, which the industry is willing to provide (see Box 11 below). Glaxo Wellcome and SmithKline Beecham make no bones about it: if use of their anti-infective products were restricted beyond a certain point, they would place their investments somewhere else.[18]

2.15 In the USA, one of the pressures towards imprudent prescribing is fear of litigation. In United Kingdom law, a doctor who prescribes in accordance with a local policy is unlikely to be successfully sued for negligence (Davey p 156). Professor James Petrie of the University of Aberdeen described the British legal position in this area as "reassuring" (Q 674). Dr McGavock expressed himself more concerned about being sued for prescribing too much than for prescribing

---

17 *Restrictive reporting*: When a doctor sends a specimen to a laboratory for microbiological analysis and susceptibility testing, the microbiologist must decide what to report. Reporting every bacterial isolate would be unhelpful, since it would include normal flora and contaminants; the doctor is interested only in possible pathogens. Reporting the susceptibility of each isolate to every conceivable antimicrobial would be impossible; in practice, only certain susceptibilities are tested or reported. In the United Kingdom, microbiologists turn these facts of life to advantage. According to the AMM, "Reporting is tailored to what is felt to be appropriate for the individual patient and the wider context, and is often made to be concordant with the hospital's formulary and antibacterial policies".

18 GW: "The outcome will be a "deprioritisation" of this area in favour of others" (p 407). SKB: "Inappropriate restrictions...would of necessity cause companies to invest their research effort in other, more profitable, therapeutic areas" (p 475).

Box 3

FORMULARIES, POLICIES AND GUIDELINES:
EXAMPLES OF GOOD PRACTICE

Grampian Formulary

The Grampian Formulary has broad ownership in both hospital and general practice and vigorous monitoring by ward pharmacists and Health Board Prescribing Advisers. Professor Petrie claims that it achieves GP concurrence or compliance of 90–96 per cent (QQ 648, 672, 684). It is commended by the Scottish Microbiology Association (p 471).

Scottish Intercollegiate Guidelines Network (SIGN)

SIGN (Q 663) is a wide group of professionals and others who are working together to produce evidence-based guidelines for a range of conditions. There are formal procedures for proposing a guideline, prioritising projects, literature reviews, grading of evidence and recommendations, and critical appraisal. 21 guidelines have been published, on paper and on the Internet, and 48 are in preparation; infectious diseases are rising up SIGN's list of priorities. Putting the guidelines into practice has involved groups of GPs, associations of patients, and newspapers; and the Royal Colleges and the Scottish Council for Postgraduate Dental and Medical Education use them in the process of accreditation for training. There are arrangements for audit and feedback. Professor Petrie emphasized the importance of local "ownership", and of implementation; "simply sending out a guideline is a waste of time" (Q 664).

PRODIGY

PRODIGY (Prescribing Rationally with Decision Support in General Practice) is a project to develop an electronic guideline (or "decision support") system, intended for use on a GP's desktop computer. Dr Davey commended PRODIGY (Q 250). So did the RCGP (p 167, Q 290); they told us that PRODIGY is being piloted in 200 practices with funding from the Department of Health, and that other similar systems are under development. The Department observe that guidance delivered through PRODIGY is "adjusted to local conditions to reinforce local policies"; and that computer prescribing systems are in use in some hospitals (p 344).

too little (Q 642).

Rapid testing

2.16 Susceptibility testing by the standard methods takes 48 hours; the whole process, from the doctor taking the specimen to receiving the result, may take longer. In the meantime, the doctor must prescribe empirically, and may prescribe inappropriately. Many witnesses have put it to us that the cause of prudent use would be much advanced by more rapid testing. According to the ABPI, rapid testing for routine infections is on the way. "People are working on it, and it will become available in due course"—perhaps in 5–10 years (Q 341). SmithKline Beecham call on the Government to support technology development, possibly through the EU (p 485).

2.17 The PHLS agreed that faster testing would be helpful (Q 109). "Genotypic" tests, which use the polymerase chain reaction (PCR) to examine the isolate's DNA, are already in use. However, these "will not replace the existing methods entirely", because they are expensive, and because they answer only one question at a time. Professor Roger Finch of the University of Nottingham believes that the expense of genotypic testing for the wide range of infections encountered in general practice will be prohibitive (Q 385). Dr Davey sounded a further note of caution (QQ 269–271): even if rapid analysis were available, it would say only that a certain organism was present, not that it was necessarily the cause of the disease.

2.18 Even without faster tests, the process could be speeded up if results could be reported electronically. The RCGP told us that systems to do this exist already (Q 294). The recent NHS White Paper *The new NHS* (Cm 3807) indicates that one immediate application envisaged for the projected "NHSnet", linking all hospitals and GP practices, is to be transmission of test results (paragraph 1.12).

Prescription checking and control

2.19 A hospital formulary may incorporate controls, whereby certain agents may be prescribed only with certain levels of authority. According to the AMM, "Recent evidence from the USA shows that it is possible by considerable effort (prior approval from an infection specialist for the use of an antibacterial from a restricted list) to influence prescribing without adversely affecting clinical outcomes and with improvements in the sensitivities of bacteria" (p 10).

2.20 According to the Department of Health (p 344), although routine prescribing of antimicrobials in hospitals is done by junior doctors, "Access to non-routine agents is restricted through the hospital pharmacy", and in most hospitals pharmacists visit the wards every day to check prescriptions and advise.[19] However the PHLS clinical audit project found that practice in this respect, in hospitals in England and Wales, "varied greatly"; and Dr Davey, as a hospital consultant, admitted that prescribing by junior doctors at night is often not reviewed by senior staff in the morning (QQ 245, 268). He suggested that there might be a role here for senior nurses.

2.21 Senior practitioners whom we met in Boston disagreed as to the appropriate level of control. Dr Sherwood Gorbach favoured requiring that every prescription for a drug associated with a resistance problem be accompanied by a "chit" giving the reason for prescribing. Dr Anton Medeiros considered that this would restrict professional freedom to a degree unacceptable in the USA; he believed that, if surveillance was thorough and its findings were properly communicated, doctors would moderate their practice voluntarily. See Appendix 6.

2.22 In general practice, there is a long and strong tradition of clinical freedom and responsibility. Dr McGavock considered (QQ 650, 657–660, and p 300) that liberty has degenerated into licence, and that the seriousness of the threat to the effectiveness of antimicrobials justifies extreme measures. He recommended that GPs should be prohibited from prescribing specific new, expensive, broad-spectrum antibiotics without first receiving microbiological advice. Professor Petrie considered this to be unaffordable and impractical. Dr McGavock acknowledged that it would be expensive, but insisted that it was a price worth paying to prolong the "antimicrobial era".

Pharmaceutical licensing

2.23 It would in principle be possible for a licensing authority, considering a new application, to turn it down on the basis that the new drug, though effective, was no more so than drugs already on the market, and was more likely to induce resistance. This is not however the usual approach. Dr Ross Taylor of the RCGP told us (Q 283), "I think the fundamental problem is that in this country medicines are licensed on the basis of effectiveness, not comparative effectiveness. So, if an antibiotic is licensed, a company can quite legitimately...promote that medicine...whether or not there is another antibiotic already available that might be better". Similarly, it would in principle be possible for a licensing authority to modify or withdraw a licence if resistance induced by the drug rose to a certain level (Finch p 189). Dr McGavock recommended that certain antibiotics should be licensed for hospital use only, so that GPs could not use them at all (p 300).

19 The Hammersmith Hospital has appointed a specialist clinical pharmacist working exclusively on antimicrobials. This has led to reduced infection, and annual savings of £77,000 (DH p 345). On the general role of the hospital pharmacist, see the evidence of the Royal Pharmaceutical Society, p 461.

Pharmaceutical salesmanship

2.24 The AMM blame the increase in prescribing of antimicrobials, and the tendency to prescribe more expensive drugs where cheaper ones would do, on advertising and salesmanship by the pharmaceutical industry. The comments of the Department of Health on the increased use of ciprofloxacin and the more expensive macrolides, noted above, suggest that they agree—though in oral evidence, the Chief Medical Officer deprecated any suggestion that the industry went beyond reasonable bounds, and said that increased use of macrolides may have been due to a new indication for use (Q 789). Professor Petrie gave a startling example of promotion which he regarded as excessive: provision by a company to a community on-call service of free "starter packs" of the antibiotics co-amoxiclav (Q 654) and clarithromycin (Q 657). The AMM call for "stricter controls" to restrain "over-zealous promotion"; so did Dr Rosamund Williams of WHO (Q 127).

2.25 Dr Mayon-White considers pharmaceutical salesmanship an "important influence" on GP prescribing, but not necessarily a bad one: "it can be a collaborative process in setting policies and getting educational messages across" (Q 158). For this to happen, he says, health authorities and doctors must be "in control of the process". The RCGP likewise declined to condemn pharmaceutical marketing outright (Q 282); they consider it necessary and useful, and believe that GPs are able to retain control. The ABPI observe that their members' marketing is governed by a code of practice administered by an independent body; they consider that the pressure on GPs to prescribe comes more from patients (see below) and from lack of time than from the industry (Q 333).

Over-the-counter (OTC) antibiotics

2.26 In the United Kingdom at present, generally speaking, systemic antibiotics (i.e. taken internally, as opposed to "topical") are licensed as "POM": i.e. prescription-only medicines, available only on prescription from a doctor, dentist or veterinary surgeon (not from a nurse-prescriber). There is however a general trend to deregulate medicines, moving them from POM to "P" (pharmacy); and there is discussion of treating antibiotics in this way.

2.27 The RCGP believe that there is pressure for OTC antibiotics from consumers and from industry. However they have no doubt that OTC availability would mean more use, and they consider it possible that this would mean more resistance. Therefore, "We do not think it is a good idea" (Q 306).[20] Neither does Professor Petrie (Q 659). The ABPI are "generally opposed" to OTC antibiotics, with the possible exception of treatments for uncomplicated lower urinary tract infection (cystitis) (p 177, Q 338). They object because pharmacists do not have the necessary training or suitable premises for the confidential consultations which would sometimes be needed to advise customers on the right choice of medicine, nor access to the microbiology services which would sometimes be needed for diagnosis; and because the imprudent use which contributes to resistance would probably increase.

2.28 Professor Finch (p 186, QQ 364–376), who is a member of the Committee on Safety of Medicines and co-chairman of a BSAC working party on OTC antibiotics, told us that the pressure to deregulate the supply of antibiotics comes not just from industry, but from the regulators themselves, in particular at EU level. He explained that what is under consideration is not a free-for-all, but OTC supply of single doses or short courses for particular indications. In his view, much depends on what drugs are to be deregulated, and for what conditions; he too identified cystitis as one which "seems to be reasonable at first view", along with minor infections of the skin or eye.[21] It would be necessary to give pharmacists robust guidelines, possibly access to medical records, and perhaps a surveillance role. OTC antibiotics would make commercial sense only if they resulted

---

[20] The RCGP's memorandum (p 167) said, "In principle...we would not object to the direct sale of certain antibiotics". They admitted under oral examination that they would object, up to the point where the Medicines Control Agency licensed antibiotics OTC, at which point "We would have to go along with that" (Q 306).

[21] Cp Royal Pharmaceutical Society p 463.

in increased use; but this would not necessarily mean more resistance, and might even mean less, if P medicines with a lower tendency to induce resistance took market share from POM drugs with a higher tendency. He concludes that more research and consideration is needed before any major change.

2.29 One systemic antimicrobial is already available OTC in the United Kingdom: the antifungal fluconazole, sold in a one-capsule course for *Candida vaginitis*. In Spain and Greece fluconazole is available OTC, and seems to have given rise to significant resistance. According to Professor Finch, "In the United Kingdom there is no evidence to date that the use in the community of a single capsule for *Candida vaginitis* is associated with resistance" (Q 375); but this may be because no survey has been undertaken. According to Dr David Denning of the University of Manchester (p 402), fluconazole-resistance in Candida is now common, but the causes are "not known entirely"; any effects of OTC supply are "not being studied".

2.30 The Department of Health drew to our attention the concern of the Medical Devices Agency about wound dressings which incorporate antibiotics (p 345). Under EU law and the Medical Devices Regulations, there is no provision for such dressings to be POM, and they have therefore been available OTC since 1995. The Agency are concerned that uncontrolled use will give rise to resistance. However they have no evidence yet that this is happening; and they have received little support from other Member States "because many antibiotics are already available OTC in a number of EU countries and there seems to be general acceptance of this practice". As to actual OTC antibiotics, however, the Department are confident that they can hold the line. The Chief Medical Officer, Sir Kenneth Calman, has raised the issue with his EU counterparts (Q 757); he considers a ministerial decision to permit OTC availability "very unlikely" (Q 794). Under EU law, any medicine may be confined to the POM category if it presents "danger to health" if used without supervision; and Sir Kenneth assured us that "health" for this purpose included public health (p 371).

Medical education: undergraduate, postgraduate and vocational

2.31 The undergraduate medical curriculum is crowded, and several witnesses told us that it tends to devote little time to antimicrobial therapy (e.g. Petrie, McGavock Q 681—though Professor Finch disagrees, p 187).[22] This would be understandable, since oral antimicrobials are relatively easy to prescribe, being relatively non-toxic and unlikely to harm the patient directly. As the AMM put it, "antibacterials are victims of their own success". They point out that "antimicrobials are the only class of drugs the prescription of which can have adverse consequences outside individual recipients"—i.e. the selection of resistant strains. They recommend, "priority should be given by the medical profession, universities and the General Medical Council to ensuring that a definitive slot on antibacterial use is in all curricula, and that this includes not only technicalities of antibacterials but puts their use into sociological and world contexts" (p 10). Implementing this recommendation would of course involve taking time from other subjects, whose advocates would no doubt make their case with equal vigour.

Continuing professional development

2.32 In medicine as in other walks of life, one of the most effective forms of professional development is participation in teaching. In Oxfordshire, Dr Mayon-White reports, "the teaching and training practices tend to prescribe less of the expensive antibiotics—and indeed fewer antibiotics overall—than the non-teaching, non-training practices" (Q 158, cp Davey p 155 and Q 250). In the context of prescribing, another effective form of professional development is participation in the process of creating local formularies and policies (Petrie Q 679).

2.33 Not every doctor can be a trainer or policy-maker; and various ways have been found to deliver professional development to the wider medical community. Dr Jeremy Grimshaw of the

22 Professor David Greenwood, of Nottingham University Hospital, believes that his department "may be unique" in giving third-year medical students a two-week module on antimicrobial therapy (p 410).

Health Services Research Unit at the University of Aberdeen gave us an overview drawn from the findings of the Cochrane Collaboration on Effective Professional Practice, of which he is the co-ordinating editor (Q 672). He indicated that there are no "magic bullets"; which interventions are most effective at changing behaviour depends on the behaviour in question, and on the context (e.g. hospital or general practice), and best results are obtained by intervening in several ways at once. Dr Grimshaw's findings may be crudely summarised as follows:

(i) *Passive dissemination*, using literature and lectures: in itself, ineffective;

(ii) *Interactive workshops*: more effective;

(iii) *Audit and feedback*: effective, though the changes achieved may be modest;

(iv) *Educational outreach*, whereby trainers visit professionals individually: "very promising";

(v) *Local opinion leaders* raising standards by example: "much touted", but requires further research (Q 683).

We have received further evidence about (iii) and (iv), as follows.

Audit and feedback

2.34 GPs may already opt to receive detailed information ("PACT" data) on their own prescribing from the PPA; and some may have access to additional information from their own IT system. The AMM, who recommend wider use of formularies and policies, call for these to be supported by audit (p 10).[23] They acknowledge that audit is especially difficult in the isolated conditions of general practice; on the other hand, GPs are ahead of hospitals in computerising their records of diagnosis and prescription. They acknowledge that the cost to the NHS of the staff and IT required for a proper system of audit would be high; and they assess the impact, even after 5–10 years, as "Some effect, but not major". Professor Petrie is an advocate of audit (Q 663): "By doing audit of what people are doing, you can get the 'outliers' and bring them into the middle group of prescribers voluntarily. If you start going out with guns and statutory controls, people hide." Box 4 gives examples of good practice in this area which have come to our notice.

Educational outreach

2.35 Dr Grimshaw defined educational outreach thus: "This is where you have a professional, often a pharmacist, going to visit a general practice or hospital to give a number of very selective messages about good prescribing behaviour, which often use the marketing techniques of the pharmaceutical industry, to try and identify the specific barriers to the behaviour they want to happen, and modify their message based on these barriers and reinforce that message throughout that contact". He mentioned that the Department of Health is currently funding a large-scale trial of this method, expected to report in 1999 (QQ 672, 683). The USA is ahead of the United Kingdom in this field: see Box 5.

Educating the public

2.36 One major factor affecting the prescribing behaviour of GPs is the expectations of their patients[24]—or GPs' perception of patients' expectations, which is not necessarily the same thing.[25] Patients' expectations are not uniform; according to Dr Grimshaw, they "vary across different areas, socio-economic groups and cultures" (p 301).

---

23 So do the British Pharmacological Society (p 386).

24 For eloquent accounts of this problem from the front line, see the evidence of the Osborne Practice in Southsea (p 440) and Dr John Sterland (p 526).

25 "Doctors tend to overestimate the patient's desire for a prescription"—RCGP Q 297, cp Grimshaw Q 674.

Box 4

PRESCRIBING AUDIT AND FEEDBACK: EXAMPLES OF GOOD PRACTICE

Northern Ireland—COMPASS

Dr McGavock told us about COMPASS—Computerised On-line Monthly Prescribing Analysed for Science and Stewardship (p 281, Q 635). COMPASS is an evidence-based, computerised prescribing interrogation system, run by the Drug Utilisation Research Unit of The Queen's University, Belfast. "COMPASS compares each practice's prescribing every month in Northern Ireland against best practice and it then prints a clear report showing the ways in which the doctors did prescribe and recommends changes to improve the quality of their prescribing". For a cost of £2 per copy, COMPASS typically identifies possible savings of 15 per cent. "COMPASS is taken to every practice annually by the Area Prescribing Advisers, for detailed discussion, but fundholding practices often request this document quarterly, to drive their cost-effectiveness efforts. COMPASS has saved over £11m in Northern Ireland in the past three years, but could save up to £25m annually, if fully utilised, with a striking improvement in the quality of medical treatment". In the first quarter of 1997, 60 non-fund-holding GPs saved £1.23m using COMPASS, backed up with lectures and visits. Dr McGavock finds the results of COMPASS overall "disappointing". He believes that, if it is to change behaviour significantly, such a system requires to be backed up by educational outreach, and by some direct "incentive", e.g. such that a proportion of the money saved on drugs is returned to the practice (QQ 638, 684).

Oxfordshire

Dr Mayon-White told us (p 111) that Oxfordshire Health Authority has begun a programme to improve antibiotic use in general practice. Guidelines have been issued to GPs, recommending first-choice empirical treatments for various infections. The guidelines are supported by prescription monitoring; results are fed back to GPs in general by means of a newsletter, and to individual practices through visits by the Authority's Medical Adviser.

2.37 It may not be the case that people in poorer communities have a higher expectation of receiving antibiotics. Rather, it may be that GPs in such communities are more pressed for time, and therefore inclined to prescribe rather than explain. However a GP under pressure of time may do various things to terminate the consultation besides prescribing. First, he may simply say No: Dr Grimshaw cited evidence from a randomised trial that this reduces the likelihood that the patient will attend again with the same complaint (Q 674). Saying No is not always easy: Dr Grimshaw recommended training for GPs in communication skills (p 301). Dr Davey mentioned two alternative approaches (Q 273): give the patient an information leaflet; or say, "I do not think you need an antibiotic, but if you want to get a prescription you can come back any time, you do not have to make another appointment". Of the latter approach, he commented, "Most of the people who were given that option did not come and get the antibiotics". Dr Taylor of the RCGP mentioned another: a delayed-action prescription, for use if symptoms persist. "The result of that is that many patients do not in fact take the prescription" (Q 303); this strategy is also known to reduce the rate of follow-up appointments.

2.38 Rather than waiting until the patient is in the surgery, the professions may take the message of prudent use out to the public at large. The AMM recommend that the health and education departments, the health professions and the media should all do more to convey the message (p 11). Dr Mayon-White similarly calls for public education; he recommends that health authorities' health education departments should prepare material for schools, while adult education should be delivered through the media (QQ 159–163).

Box 5

EDUCATIONAL OUTREACH IN THE USA

Dr Jerry Avorn of Harvard Medical School is a world expert on educational outreach. His approach is modelled on that of the pharmaceutical industry. He began with focus groups of physicians. These revealed two groups of doctors: some who overprescribe out of ignorance; and others who consciously overprescribe in order to satisfy their patients. For the second group, like Dr Schwartz, he provides "paper placebos". For the first, he sends out "academic detailmen": pharmacists from the medical school who meet physicians one-to-one, on the same basis as salesmen, to talk about prudent prescribing. He has shown that every $1 spent on these actions saves $2 on the drugs bill. His approach has been taken up in various places around the USA; similar approaches have been tried in various parts of the United Kingdom, and adopted nationwide in Australia. He acknowledged that some doctors require to be persuaded that prudent use is not just a euphemism for cutting costs at the expense of patient care.

Dr Ben Schwartz, of the Centers for Communicable Disease Control and Prevention (CDC) in Atlanta, has worked on educating community physicians and their patients, with a view to controlling the rise of penicillin-resistant pneumococcus. In focus groups, physicians acknowledged overusing antibiotics by as much as 50 per cent. They blamed pressure from patients, and shortage of consultation time: it is quicker to prescribe, than to explain why a prescription would be inappropriate. Dr Schwartz has therefore produced the following aids for physicians: professional information sheets; a simple patient information leaflet for the waiting room, explaining that unnecessary antibiotics are bad for the patient; a "non-prescription" form; question-and-answer sheets for parents; and a letter for parents to give to their child-carer. Pilot projects are now under way in five States; CDC is equipping the local health department to train senior doctors to disseminate the concepts and materials to their peers. Evaluation will show whether these approaches reduce inappropriate use, and whether this in turn affects the level of resistance.

2.39 The RCGP observe that GPs work within, and are to an extent constrained by, a "cultural framework" (Q 281). A GP who unilaterally defies this framework may simply lose his patients. However the culture can be changed, as in the cases of barbiturates and amphetamines. Changing the culture requires public education and consensus-building, based on evidence. In this matter, they feel, the evidence will have to be compelling: "Whether or not, and how far, antibiotic use for relief of symptoms of self-limiting illness should be limited should not be a matter for doctors to decide, but the subject of public policy. In a context in which antibiotics are much more freely used in agriculture and food production, it seems unlikely that there would be much public support for such restriction...Antibiotic use in the United Kingdom is already lower than in many other European countries; in that context it would be difficult to operate a more restrictive policy" (p 167). The RCGP observe that typically the sort of patients who are most insistent on antibiotics belong to the social groups who are hardest to reach with educational material (Q 299, cp Petrie Q 677).

Are antibiotics bad for you?

2.40 Persuading the public of the case for reduced use of antibiotics will be much easier if it can be shown that unnecessary use carries risks not only to public health in general, but also to the particular patient under treatment.[26]

[26] Like all medicines, antibiotics carry risks of direct adverse side-effects in the individual. Although antibiotics are generally safe medicines, unwanted effects do occur, mostly trivial but occasionally life-threatening. Our particular concern, however, is the relationship of antibiotic treatment to the development of resistance.

2.41 Professor Finch said (in the context of OTC antibiotics), "It is uncommon for resistance to arise in an individual receiving an antibiotic and for this to cause him/her harm" (p 189). (TB is an exception, as are viruses such as HIV.) However he went on, "Agents can affect the susceptibility of the bacteria which make up the normal flora of the skin and gastrointestinal tract. This in turn could give rise to subsequent infection in an individual". Dr Ben Schwartz of the US Centers for Communicable Disease Control and Prevention (CDC) and Dr Michael Bennish of Boston both believe they can show that previous treatment with antibiotics is a risk factor for infection with resistant strains. Dr McGavock cited evidence that, in cases of otitis media, withholding antibiotics for two to three days reduced the rate of recurrence by four fifths (QQ 659, 677).

2.42 Dr Davey also has evidence to support this proposition. "Patients with resistant organisms are more likely to have received prior antibiotic therapy than are controls [i.e. patients with susceptible strains of the same organism]"—though, he admits, "Antibiotic use may just be a marker for patients who are more ill" (p 145). Speaking in the context of the successful campaign in Iceland to bear down on penicillin-resistant pneumococci, he added, "The message that we need to get across is that most of the bacteria that live in our bodies do not do us any harm, and if you eliminate them with antibiotics then you allow the bad guys in" (Q 262; cp Q 236, pp 146, 154). He went so far as to say, "Germs are good for you...germs are part of your environment" (Q 274); he admitted that this is "probably not something that people understand".

2.43 The ABPI observe that effects on the gut flora are checked as part of the process of licensing a new antimicrobial. "Whilst it is true that there are occasional changes in gut flora which are limited to the duration of treatment, generally speaking you find that the gut flora returns to normal quickly after the antibiotics are stopped" (Q 331).

2.44 If antibiotics do even slight collateral damage, then it would plainly be better not to use them in situations where they can do no good (e.g. the minor viral infections which Dr Davey believes account for more than half of GPs' prescriptions—Q 265). More difficult are situations where antibiotics do a little good, which must then be weighed against the possibility of harm. The RCGP draw attention to the major grey area in general practice: the use of antibiotics to relieve the symptoms of self-limiting illness such as sore throat, bronchitis and otitis media. They concede that there may be a case for limiting use in such cases on public health grounds, but they insist that such use does have direct benefit (p 166). The ABPI, on the other hand, regard prescribing antibiotics for "the majority of sore throats", or for "a banal, self-limiting, mild condition, e.g. an upper respiratory tract infection", as "irresponsible" (p 176).

2.45 Tessa Jowell MP, the Minister for Public Health, was firmly of the view that the public must not be warned off antibiotics. For her, the issue crystallised around meningitis: nothing must be said to deter parents, in particular, from contacting their doctor at once if they suspected meningitis in their child. She acknowledged that it was difficult to convey the message of appropriate use of antibiotics in a way which was balanced and not confusing; but, she insisted, "We do not want patients to think that antimicrobials are dangerous for the individual...; they are among the safest medicines" (Q 759). The Chief Medical Officer suggested that the problem could be addressed by acknowledging that what was appropriate varied from case to case: for instance, what was appropriate for a young child with a fever was not necessarily appropriate for a middle-aged man with a cold (Q 761).

Compliance

2.46 It is usual practice for patients receiving antibiotics to be instructed to "complete the course". Yet the quality of evidence on which the recommended duration of antibiotic treatment is based varies, in fact, greatly from case to case. For some infections, of which tuberculosis is the most notable example, the type and duration of treatment needed to cure the patient (and to prevent resistance in those few patients who are not cured) has been well authenticated by numerous controlled trials. For others, including the many respiratory infections, such as bronchitis, pneumonia, sinusitis and otitis media, which constitute the most frequent occasions of antibiotic use, the optimum duration of courses of treatment is still surprisingly ill-founded. International comparisons reveal these uncertainties vividly, particularly in otitis media, bacterial endocarditis and urinary tract infection (Griffin p 548). There is certainly no virtue in completing the course if the infection was not in fact present in the first place (Davey Q 268), or if the prescribed course was longer than necessary to cure the infection and completing the course only prolongs the selective pressure on the commensal flora.

2.47 Whether or not the particular recommendations for duration of treatment are well-founded, however, it is clear that compliance with prescribing recommendations is hard to achieve and that non-compliance with treatment can contribute to resistance, especially in the case of tuberculosis and sexually-transmitted infections. The Royal Pharmaceutical Society has addressed this problem in a valuable document entitled *From Compliance to Concordance* (March 1997). The RCGP observe that compliance can be encouraged by drug and regimen design, and by patient information, on which there is recent EU legislation which they support (p 167). The ABPI are "particularly keen" on improving compliance by means of new formulations (p 176, Q 347); and they support the Patient Pack Initiative on patient information.

CHAPTER 3 PRUDENT USE IN ANIMALS

3.1 It may be that as much as half of all antimicrobial usage by volume takes place outside human medicine (PHLS Q 82; SKB p 475); and we were aware before we began our enquiry of the relevance to our topic of the use of antibiotics as growth promoters, and for prophylactic and therapeutic purposes, in animals and fish, and the use of antibiotic resistance markers in genetically modified organisms. The former is currently under consideration by a working group of the Government's Advisory Committee on the Microbiological Safety of Food (Georgala p 373, Simmons Q 437, Calman Q 769), and the latter has recently been considered by the Advisory Committee on Novel Foods and Processes (Q 437). Therefore these questions have not been the main focus of this enquiry. However, too many witnesses have brought the issue of growth promoters to our attention, to allow us to disregard it.

3.2 Antimicrobial use in livestock originated some 50 years ago when chlortetracycline fermentation waste was found to enhance the growth of poultry, pigs and other species. Intensification of livestock production was an increasing practice of the time and the use of broad spectrum antibiotics was shown to control the diseases, especially respiratory and enteric conditions, attendant on intensive production. The use of antibiotics in animals is now a significant part of the armamentarium of veterinary medicine for all species. Their use is now regulated both nationally (Medicines Act 1968) and at EU level (Directive 70/524 for feed additives, 81/851 for medicines).

Animal medicines

3.3 Antimicrobials are used in animals for the treatment of clinical disease, the larger food species and companion animals being treated individually. With intensive systems, such as poultry and pigs, individual treatment may be, and usually is, not feasible and mass oral medication is the only practical method of treatment. This may be administered in the food or more usually in the drinking water.

3.4 Prophylactic antibiotic use is applied with respect to predictable diseases or at the outbreak of a disease in a herd or flock. This is usually applied as mass medication ("metaphylaxis"). Examples are the use of medicated feed or water to prevent the emergence of disease in poultry when it is known that mycoplasma organisms are transmitted vertically through the egg to cause disease in chicks, the occurrence of respiratory problems when young animals are regrouped, colibacillosis during the post-weaning period in pigs, and "shipping fever" following transport. The case for group treatment, and for medication via water rather than food, is put succinctly in the evidence of the National Office of Animal Health (NOAH, Q 422, pp 199 and 214) and the British Poultry Meat Federation (BPMF, p 387); but some observers consider that the borderline between mass prophylaxis and growth promotion, which is crucial to the regulatory regime, is poorly delineated (e.g. SKB p 475, Bates p 378, Simmons Q 467, Soil Association p 508).

Growth promoters

3.5 The use of antimicrobial agents as growth promoters[27] has been practised for some thirty years. They improve the growth rate and efficiency of feed in cattle, pigs and poultry. Their mode of action is not fully understood; it is said to be by suppressing commensal bacteria which would divert nutrition from the animal, and by maintaining a more effective and absorptive gut lining (NOAH Q 412, p 212; BPMF p 388; Simmons p 216). Growth promoters are used at low concentrations (2.5 ppm to 50 ppm according to compound). Their use increases average daily growth and food conversion ratios by 3 per cent to 11 per cent depending on species; in financial terms, this is considered to make the difference between profit and loss.

---

27 The industry prefers the term "digestive enhancers", which more accurately reflects what these substances do (BPMF p 388); but "growth promoters" is the term in familiar usage. The growth promoting antimicrobials in use include: Carbodox, Olaquindox, Avilamycin, Avoparcin, Efrotomycin, Flavophospholipol, Oleandamycin, Spiramycin, Tylosin and Virginiamycin.

3.6 Though applied in sub-therapeutic doses, growth promoters also appear to have the effect of suppressing disease (Q 418). While antibiotics for therapeutic use are available on a prescription-only basis (POMs), growth promoters are generally available to livestock producers from food manufacturers ("Pharmacy and Merchant's List"—PML), without veterinary prescription.[28]

Human health concerns

3.7 The widespread use of antimicrobial agents as growth promoters, and the public health implications of their use, precipitated the appointment of a Committee on the Use of Antibiotics in Animal Husbandry and Veterinary Medicine (the Swann Committee: see Box 6) which in 1969 recommended banning the use of human therapeutic antibiotics as growth promoters for animals. This led to legislation. However no restriction was placed on the use of such antibiotics for therapy or prophylaxis in animal use. In 1992, the Expert Group on Animal Feedingstuffs (the Lamming Committee) recommended that prophylactic use should be "reconsidered"; the Veterinary Products Committee accordingly reconsidered it, and decided to "discourage" it, while continuing to consider each case on its merits.

3.8 Despite the Swann Report, the use of antimicrobial agents as growth promoters continues to generate criticism that they are used for purely economic reasons and as substitutes for good husbandry and hygiene, and that because of the risk to human health they should be banned (e.g. SKB p 475, Soil Association p 505), or at any rate restricted (e.g. Simmons Q 451). According to the BPMF (p 388), "The only antibacterials authorised as digestive enhancers are ones that are not used, or related to those used, in human medicine. Antibacterials which are known or suspected of causing resistance in human bacteria are not used". However avoparcin and virginiamycin would appear to be important exceptions: see below, Enterococci. Moreover, an agent reserved for animals today may be discovered tomorrow to have clinical applications in man; and resistance by the particular mechanism of efflux can act on highly diverse molecular classes, so that treatment with an animal agent might well give rise to cross-resistance to an unrelated agent used in man (SKB p 475).

3.9 In the course of our inquiry, the WHO convened a major multidisciplinary meeting on this subject.[29] Its report concluded, "Antimicrobial use leads to the selection of resistant forms of bacteria in the ecosystem of use. This will occur with all uses including treatment, prophylaxis and growth promotion...Low-level, long-term exposure to antimicrobials may have a greater selective potential than short-term full-dose therapeutic use". The meeting recommended prohibition of growth promoters which are "used in human therapeutics, or known to select for cross-resistance to antimicrobials used in human medicine"; and "a systematic approach towards replacing growth-promoting antimicrobials with safer non-antimicrobial alternatives". The Chief Medical Officer acknowledged the importance of the WHO meeting, and said, "The area is one of significant concern" (Q 769). Dr Robin Bywater of Pfizer, who attended the WHO meeting, told us that the industry would be "fully supportive" of reduced reliance on antimicrobial growth promoters, "if such products can be replaced by effective alternatives" such as probiotics[30] (Q 395).

3.10 The animal health and welfare and environmental benefits of growth promoters have been clearly delineated by NOAH (QQ 406–421), the BPMF (p 388) and UKASTA (p 533), and are illustrated by the experience of Sweden in trying to do without them (see below). Antimicrobial resistance in diseases affecting the animals themselves is of welfare and economic concern in animal production, but NOAH does not see it as a major problem in that context (p 212). What matters for our purposes is the potential of animal-derived resistant organisms and their genes

---

28 The regulatory regime for animal feed is described in the evidence of the Veterinary Medicines Directorate (p 565) and the UK Agricultural Supply Trade Association (UKASTA, p 529).

29 Medical Impact of the Use of Antimicrobials in Food Animals, Berlin, 13–17 October 1997.

30 Probiotics work on the principle that harmful micro-organisms in the alimentary tract may be kept at low levels by displacing them with benign or beneficial organisms, as opposed to destroying them with antibiotics.

Box 6

THE SWANN REPORT

The Joint Committee on the use of Antibiotics in Animal Husbandry and Veterinary Medicine, chaired by Professor M M Swann, was appointed jointly by Health and Agriculture Ministers in July 1968. Its report (Cmnd 4190) was issued in November 1969.

The Swann Report concluded that "the administration of antibiotics to farm livestock, particularly at sub-therapeutic levels, poses certain hazards to human and animal health"; in particular it had led to resistance in enteric bacteria of animal origin. This resistance was transmissible to other bacteria (it had been the discovery that this might be so, followed by an epidemic of resistant *S. typhimurium* in 1963–65, which prompted Ministers to appoint the Committee); and enteric bacteria were transferable from animals to man.

It therefore recommended that only antibiotics which "have little or no application as therapeutic agents in man or animals and will not impair the efficacy of a prescribed therapeutic drug or drugs through the development of resistant strains of organisms" should be usable for growth promotion. The Report named the following antibiotics, which were then in use for growth promotion, as unsuitable for such use: chlortetracycline, oxytetracycline, penicillin, tylosin (a macrolide related to erythromycin) and the sulphonamides. The Government largely accepted these recommendations.

The Report recommended that a single advisory committee, constituted under the Medicines Act 1968, "should have overall responsibility for the whole field of use of antibiotics and related substances whether in man, animals, food preservation, or for other purposes". It also recommended research into alternative means of growth promotion; and improved surveillance and epidemiology of diseases common to animals and man.

passing to humans, either via direct contact with animals[31] or through the consumption of food or water.

3.11 Antimicrobial residues in food of animal origin (regulated by acceptable maximum residue levels—MRLs) are considered to be a low risk (NOAH p 200, BPMF p 390, UKASTA p 530). The Soil Association suggest that therefore the Veterinary Medicines Directorate (VMD) and the Veterinary Laboratories Agency (VLA) should pay less attention to residues, and more to resistance (p 501).

3.12 There is a marked discrepancy of opinion about the link between antibiotic use in animals and resistance in man. The argument is being conducted in conditions of some heat[32] and inadequate light. Dr Norman Simmons, a Consultant Microbiologist and a member of both ACMSF and ACNFP, told us that United Kingdom veterinary medicine does not look for resistance (Q 438).[33] NOAH responded (p 212) that the pharmacovigilance section of the VMD, and the VLA, are generally aware of the resistance pattern in the United Kingdom; but they admitted that there is "a shortage of data gathered in a consistent manner which would allow thorough evaluation of changes in [animal] gut flora over a period of years" and their relationship to human infection. Surveillance in this area is generally agreed to be less than optimal. The report of the WHO meeting stresses the need for international action to produce better information as to the prevalence and

---

31 Including companion animals, ie horses and pets (BPMF p 388).

32 See for example the tone of the supplementary memorandum from NOAH, and the divergence between the WHO press release following the Berlin meeting and the final report of the meeting (WHO Q 135, NOAH p 213).

33 The British Veterinary Association call for epidemiological surveys in this area as a "key priority" (p 393).

spread of resistance in zoonotic bacteria,[34] using monitoring networks such as the EU's ENTERNET (formerly SALM-NET, developed by PHLS).

3.13 It is important to recognise what are the hazards presented by antimicrobial resistance in animals to human health. The first is the transfer of resistant zoonotic pathogens. The second is the selection of antimicrobial-resistant bacteria which are not pathogenic for man, but which may transfer their resistance via plasmids to human commensal and pathogenic bacteria, which may later cause resistant disease.

3.14 As NOAH rightly observe (p 199), many problem pathogens, e.g. MRSA, have nothing to do with animals or food; and much of the food-poisoning which is the cause of widespread concern both here and in the USA is not caused by resistant organisms. However, animal antibiotics are implicated in the rise of resistance in some strains of Salmonella, Campylobacter, Enterococcus, and *E. coli*; we consider each of these below.

Salmonella

3.15 The recent history of Salmonella in the United Kingdom, as told by the PHLS (p 56), is closely related to the history of antibiotics for animals. The Swann enquiry of 1969 was precipitated by an epidemic of multi-resistant *S. typhimurium DT 29* in cattle and man. Following the Swann report and the withdrawal of growth promoters related to human antibiotics such as chloramphenicol, levels of DT 29 rapidly subsided. A second wave of multi-resistant *S. typhimurium* (DT 204, DT 193 and DT 204c) ensued from 1975; this followed the introduction of some of the affected antimicrobials into calf husbandry, and provided "the first conclusive evidence" of a veterinary antibiotic (apramycin) giving rise to resistance to a human antibiotic (gentamicin). Since 1990 there has been a third wave of multi-resistant *S. typhimurium* (DT 104); since 1994 multi-drug resistance has also increased in *S. virchow*, less prevalent than *S. typhimurium* but more invasive in man, and in *S. hadar*.[35] Substantial increases in resistance to the fluoroquinolone ciprofloxacin in *S. hadar* and *S. virchow*, and in multi-resistance in *S. typhimurium DT 104*, followed the licensing for veterinary use of the fluoroquinolones enrofloxacin in 1993 and danofloxacin in 1996. PHLS concludes, "The use of fluoroquinolones and trimethoprim in food animals has contributed to the development of resistance to these antibiotics in zoonotic Salmonellas" (cp QQ 85–88).

3.16 According to Dr Simmons, "The appearance of ciprofloxacin resistance in strains from man coincided with the approval of enrofloxacin for veterinary use in the United Kingdom, and some microbiologists feel strongly that it is a consequence of it" (p 220). Dr Janice Bates of Worthing Hospital is one of them (p 378; cp BMA p 382). The report of the WHO meeting concludes that there is "direct evidence" that antimicrobial use in animals selects for resistant Salmonella serotypes, which have been transmitted to man, and "particular concern" about fluoroquinolone-resistance. Experts at PHLS, and others both in the United Kingdom and in the USA, believe that the fluoroquinolones should be used exclusively for treating human disease.[36]

3.17 Mr Peter Watson of Bayer, speaking for NOAH, offered us some evidence on the other side (Q 424). First, some of the strains recorded in the laboratory as being resistant were still susceptible to treatment in clinical conditions.[37] Second, a recent survey in Northern Ireland found no Salmonella of bovine origin resistant to fluoroquinolones, despite widespread use of fluoroquinolones in cattle in the Republic of Ireland since 1986. NOAH believes that

---

34 Bacteria found in animals and transmissible to man.

35 Resistant strains of the Salmonella responsible for most human food-poisoning in the United Kingdom, *S. enteritidis*, have throughout this period remained rare (BPMF p 389). Most cases of Salmonella do not require antibiotic treatment; but antibiotics are needed by vulnerable patients, and when Salmonella gives rise to bacteraemia. So resistance is of concern in human medicine; also, resistant strains are harder to eradicate in animals (Soil Association p 506).

36 We understand that the WHO and the FDA are to meet in June 1998 to discuss this.

37 "This may not be the case" (Piddock p 444).

fluoroquinolone resistance in Salmonella in the rest of the United Kingdom may be on the wane (p 212), and that the level of resistance to apramycin is "ultra-low" and "of no clinical significance" (p 211).

Campylobacter

3.18 Campylobacters are the most common cause of food-poisoning in the United Kingdom. According to the WHO report, "Following the introduction of fluoroquinolones for use in poultry [notably enrofloxacin, licensed in the United Kingdom in 1993] there has been a dramatic rise in the prevalence of fluoroquinolone-resistant *Campylobacter jejuni* isolated in live poultry, poultry meat and from infected humans. Moreover, prior to any use in poultry, no resistant strains were reported in individuals with no previous exposure to quinolones. Fluoroquinolone-resistant *C. jejuni* has been associated with therapeutic failures in humans".

3.19 Dr Bates, citing evidence from the Netherlands, claims that ciprofloxacin-resistance in Campylobacter is "secondary" to use of enrofloxacin in poultry (p 378; cp Piddock p 445). The BPMF acknowledge the evidence from the Netherlands to this effect, and also evidence from Spain (p 389); they blame the situation on a lack of control on the use of fluoroquinolones in poultry in those countries, and they acknowledge a lack of data on this problem in the United Kingdom.

Enterococci

3.20 Enterococci have natural resistance to numerous antibiotics, and cause serious infections in hospitalised immune-impaired patients. Infection with enterococci resistant to the glycopeptide vancomycin (VRE) is almost untreatable (PHLS p 44). The report of the WHO meeting expresses concern at the possibility of "increased dissemination of glycopeptide resistance genes to *Enterococcus faecalis* and their spread to other gram-positive organisms, particularly to MRSA for which vancomycin is the drug of last resort". According to the PHLS, "The public health and economic consequences of [such spread] would be catastrophic".[38]

3.21 Avoparcin is a glycopeptide, which has been used as a growth promoter since 1975. WHO bluntly state that the use of avoparcin as a growth promoter in animal husbandry "has contributed" to the reservoir of transferable resistance genes to glycopeptides, including vancomycin, in the commensal enterococci of animals, and that these can reach humans via the food chain. Whether resistant strains derived from animals are the same as the resistant strains which cause human disease is a matter of current scientific controversy.[39] The EU Scientific Committee for Animal Nutrition (SCAN) considered the matter in 1995, decided that the case was not proven, and recommended further research; but in 1996 the European Union decided to suspend use of avoparcin altogether.[40]

3.22 The PHLS (p 44) tell us that there is "considerable evidence" that VRE may spread to humans via the food chain, and that "several studies have implicated" avoparcin. The new antibiotic Synercid[41] is the PHLS's best hope as a treatment for multi-resistant enterococci; but resistance to Synercid may have been induced already by use of the related growth promoter virginiamycin, used in pigs, poultry and cattle. PHLS recommend extensive further study of the relative contribution of clinical antibiotics and animal growth promoters to the selective pressure on enterococci, including (a) molecular typing, to establish whether resistant strains found in people and animals are the same, (b) characterisation of resistance genes, and of their capacity to transfer between

---

38 Cp Amyes and Young, p 375, on VRE and VRSA.

39 One of those who believes that the strains are distinct is Professor Mark Casewell, whom we met at King's College Hospital: see Appendix 5.

40 Dr Johan Vanhemelrijk, Secretary-General of the European Federation of Animal Health (FEDESA), commented, "The Commission Directive is based on the absence of the disproof of risk; I think that is a strange way of making law" (Q 396). SKB support the ban, as "a precautionary and protective measure in the current climate of doubt" (p 475). NOAH considers the "precautionary principle" to be "ill-judged" (p 212); the BPMF acknowledge the force of the precautionary principle, but consider the ban unwarranted even on that basis (p 390). The only Member State to vote against the ban was the United Kingdom (Simmons p 219).

41 Trade name for a combination of the streptogramins quinupristin and dalfopristin, which may be licensed soon.

enterococci in animals and those in man, and (c) investigation of the agents being used instead of avoparcin, to find out whether they are continuing to select for cross-resistance to glycopeptides. They call also for surveillance of VRE in the community and the food chain; at present what data there are come from hospitals.

3.23 We put to NOAH the question of virginiamycin and Synercid. Dr Bywater replied that, though virginiamycin has been used in animals for thirty years, the enterococcus which is the target organism remains "almost entirely susceptible". However according to Dr Bates (p 379), "Evidence emerging from the United Kingdom, Germany and the Netherlands shows that resistance to Synercid in clinical strains already exists".

3.24 Defenders of avoparcin (e.g. NOAH, p 200, Q 397, BPMF p 390) point out that VRE is common in the USA, despite the fact that avoparcin has never been permitted there as a growth promoter. Dr Bates (p 379) accepts that VRE in the USA is probably due to human use of vancomycin, which is greater there than in Europe. However, some experts whom we met in the USA believe that there is substantial illegal use of avoparcin in the livestock industry, and that because of the global nature of food transport and travel there are opportunities to import vancomycin-resistant organisms (cp Simmons Q 448, Soil Association p 506). NOAH also observe that VRE is found in horses, for which avoparcin is not used (QQ 396, 401); and the BPMF point out that in Denmark, where avoparcin was widely used, VRE in humans is "virtually unknown" (p 390).

E. coli

3.25 Certain *E. coli* are food-borne pathogens but most are susceptible to antimicrobials at present. However, the development of antimicrobial resistance in *E. coli* is of concern since there is a high propensity to disseminate antimicrobial-resistant genes.

3.26 Dr Laura Piddock of the University of Birmingham has studied acquisition of ciprofloxacin-resistance by *E. coli*; she believes, "The primary exposure is likely to be in an animal due to the veterinary use of fluoroquinolones" (p 444). According to Dr Simmons, some fluoroquinolone-resistant *E. coli* "seem to be associated with enrofloxacin usage in animals" (p 220).

Swedish experience

3.27 Sweden banned the use of antimicrobials for in-feed use without prescription in 1986. On joining the EU, Sweden received a derogation to assess the acceptability and validity of the EU's animal production model and the use of approved in-feed antimicrobial additives for meat-producing animals. However, the ban has resulted in lower production efficiency and increased costs (NOAH p 201, QQ 406–421). In no single year has the pig industry made a profit and it is at present supported by Government subsidy.

3.28 Absence of growth promoters was associated with an increase in post-weaning scour (Institute of Biology p 423), mortality and a longer growth rate. Disease control has been achieved by improved management, the licensed use of prescribed antimicrobials, and in-feed zinc oxide.[42] According to the BPMF, the Swedish experience suggests that a husbandry system without growth promoters may even use more antimicrobials in total than a conventional system, including more therapeutic agents directly related to antibiotics used in man (p 388; cp UKASTA p 531); but according to the Soil Association, overall use of antibiotics in Sweden fell by 30 per cent by 1988 and has remained low (p 504).

3.29 Though the Swedish pig industry is recognised as inefficient, the Swedish government are seeking to persuade other EU countries to follow their lead on the basis of control of health hazards to humans and consumer concerns.

[42] Zinc oxide is not favoured by environmentalists because of its ability as a heavy metal to stay in the soil.

US experience

3.30 In 1995 the US Food and Drug Administration (FDA) approved the prescription of the quinolone sarafloxacin for the prevention of pneumonia in poultry, subject to resistance monitoring up and down the food chain. Then, in 1997, a telephone call from the PHLS Laboratory of Enteric Pathogens alerted FDA to the emergence of ciprofloxacin resistance in *S. typhimurium DT104* in the United Kingdom. Since then, FDA has issued no more approvals for fluoroquinolones for animals; meanwhile, resistance to fluoroquinolones has been found in Campylobacter, though none as yet in Salmonella. FDA are using DNA fingerprinting to see whether resistance in Campylobacter can be traced to poultry and sarafloxacin. In discussion at FDA, during our visit to the USA (see Appendix 6), we were taken aback to be asked why the United Kingdom continues to approve fluoroquinolones for animal use, when the USA has stopped doing so on information from the PHLS.

Licensing regime

3.31 The Swann Report recommended that a single Government advisory committee "should have overall responsibility for the whole field of use of antibiotics and related substances whether in man, animals, food preservation, or for other purposes". This recommendation was implemented by the establishment of the Joint Committee on Antimicrobial Substances (JCAMS), as a sub-committee of the Committee for the Safety of Medicines and the Veterinary Products Committee; but JCAMS was wound up in 1980. The Soil Association (p 501) put it to us that JCAMS was not effective, and that Swann's original recommendation ought now to be implemented in full.[43]

3.32 NOAH drew our attention to a potential gap in the licensing arrangements for feed additives in the United Kingdom (p 198, QQ 403–5). Both the United Kingdom and the European Union regimes are to change as from 1 April 1998. Directive 70/524 is to be amended so as to move from approval of substances to approval of individual branded products; meanwhile the United Kingdom licensing requirements under the Medicines Act are to be revoked altogether. It will be "a number of years" before the new EU regime is fully in place; during that period, according to NOAH, there will be "a free and uncontrolled market for antibiotic growth promoters in the United Kingdom".

Aquaculture

3.33 Several of those whom we have met, in both the United Kingdom and the USA (e.g. PHLS Q 82), have suggested that we should take into account the use of antibiotics in aquaculture (fish-farming). Hitherto, fish farming has relied heavily on the use of antibiotics; and, for example, catfish farming has been associated with resistant Aeromonas and Vibrios. However, the development of a vaccine for furunculosis has resulted in a marked reduction in antibiotic use in the United Kingdom and other countries (NOAH pp 201, 212). Nevertheless, antibiotic use is substantial in Asia, and there is a resistance problem in ornamental fish (Simmons Q 461) and terrapins.

Uses of antimicrobial agents on plants

3.34 Antibiotic-resistant organisms may be found on common fruits and vegetables following the use of antibiotic sprays to control bacterial and fungal growth (Institute of Biology p 425). While there is little direct danger from eating fruit and vegetables treated in this way, the organisms could transfer their resistance to more potent human pathogens.

3.35 The bacterium *Burkholderia cepacia* is used widely for environmental purposes (biodegradation of landfill wastes), and also for enhancement of crop yields and prevention of post-harvest loss of fruit and vegetables through its antifungal properties. Dr Philip Murphy, Director of the Northern Ireland Public Health Laboratory, drew our attention to concern about its use, given its significance as a pathogen in cystic fibrosis and its resistance to all available antibiotics (p 435).

---

[43] Cp Dr R Hill (p 420), who recommends medical involvement in the licensing of veterinary drugs, and the Institute of Biology (p 422), who call for a "holistic" approach to the whole phenomenon of resistance.

Sheep: worms and scab

3.36 Dr Gerald Coles of Bristol University (p 250) expressed concern about two major parasitic infections of sheep: nematodes (worms) and sheep scab. These pose no threat to human health, but can have a serious impact on farming and on animal welfare. Nematodes resistant to all anthelmintic treatments have forced some farms to close in South Africa, and have been found in Australia and New Zealand, and in two herds of Angora goats in the United Kingdom. "The evidence is that most [United Kingdom] farmers are not yet taking the problem seriously. The problem is compounded by the fact that some of the recommendations [for controlling resistance] have never been validated in the field due to the lack of research funds." Dr Coles blames multi-resistance on over-use of anthelmintics; he considers it "most probable" that the worms have passed from goats to sheep. He recommends that all sheep grazed with Angora goats should be monitored, and that sheep carrying worms resistant to ivermectin should be banned from sale except for slaughter. The Ministry of Agriculture, Fisheries and Food (MAFF) acknowledge that the situation "merits some degree of concern" (p 551).

3.37 Until 1992 sheep scab was kept at low levels in the United Kingdom by compulsory dipping (MAFF p 551). In 1992 these controls were lifted, and since then levels of scab have risen. What is worse, resistance has emerged to both pyrethroids and organophosphates (though not yet to both together), either through inappropriate use against scab, or through the effect on undiagnosed scab of correct use against other infestations. Dr Coles paints a gloomy picture: "It is quite probable that resistance to the third group [of insecticides, i.e. ivermectin] has already developed, or will do so shortly...It is quite probable that multi-resistant mites will occur within 3-5 years. On welfare grounds this would leave only the reintroduction of the organochlorine lindane, or slaughter of the affected flock(s). If organophosphates are banned, flock slaughter may have to start within two years".

3.38 MAFF are less pessimistic (p 551). "MAFF is aware of reports on the limited existence of sheep scab mites in the United Kingdom flock which are resistant to either pyrethroid or organophosphate classes of treatment compounds. However, there is no evidence of such mites having a resistance to both pyrethroids and organophosphates. There are no recorded cases of resistance to ivermectin, the third class of treatment compound, in sheep scab mites anywhere in the world. We consider therefore that there are effective treatments currently available against sheep scab in the United Kingdom flock. The potential problem of the further development of acaricide resistance in sheep scab mites is nevertheless recognised and MAFF is funding research into the factors which are involved, together with surveillance methodology, and possible alternatives in sheep scab control."

3.39 The previous Government went back somewhat on the deregulation of 1992, and made it compulsory to treat flocks visibly affected by scab and illegal to move them in the mean time (Sheep Scab Order 1997, S.I. 1997 No. 968). However, according to Dr Coles, this is not enough. "Firstly, sub-clinical scab cannot be diagnosed, so scab will still be spread. Secondly, without rapid sensitive tests for resistance, farmers will not know if they are using a fully effective product...Without diagnosis of the resistance status of outbreaks, incompletely effective treatments may be used, resulting in further sub-clinical scab and dissemination of the resistance mites."

3.40 MAFF reply, "The objective of the Sheep Scab Order is not to eradicate the sheep scab mite but to facilitate the control of clinical disease by sheep farmers" (p 552). Sub-clinical disease, and the effectiveness of treatments, are not the concern of the Order.

3.41 The British sheep industry is the biggest in the EU; and Dr Coles considers that resistance in nematodes and scab mites is imperilling its future. He calls for recognition of the problem by Government and farmers (Q 562); for surveillance (Q 535), and for research into how resistance arises, how to detect it and how to avoid it (QQ 541, 564; see MAFF p 551); for voluntary or compulsory certification of health when sheep are sold (QQ 545, 550); and for vigorous programmes of eradication while effective treatments remain.

Antibiotic-resistance marker genes in genetically-modified organisms

3.42 When a genetic modification is made to an organism using techniques of bioengineering, it is usual to incorporate a "marker" to indicate whether the modification has been a success. One suitable form of marker is a gene which codes for resistance to an antibiotic: the modified organism can then be exposed to the antibiotic, and if it resists then the modification has worked.

3.43 It has been suggested in some quarters that there is a risk that resistance genes incorporated into genetically-modified organisms as markers may somehow confer resistance on pathogens. This possibility has been considered by the Government's Advisory Committee on Novel Foods and Processes (ACNFP); the EU Scientific Committees for Food, and for Animal Nutrition (SCAN); and by the WHO and the FAO. The consensus is that the risk of transfer is very small, and that even if it were to happen the effect on the overall resistance picture would be marginal. There has been however a disagreement between the ACNFP and SCAN over a genetically-modified maize containing a marker gene for β-lactam resistance in *E. coli*; the story is told in the evidence of Dr Simmons, a member of the ACNFP, who considers that the EU set an unfortunate precedent by allowing the maize to be imported (p 221, Q 469; cp Monsanto p 434).

3.44 Of the many witnesses who have expressed to us their grave concern about the issue of antibiotic resistance, none has pointed to biotechnology as a contributory factor[44]; therefore we have not gone into this matter in detail.

44 Though the Institute of Biology express concern (p 424).

CHAPTER 4 INFECTION CONTROL

4.1 As resistance to antimicrobials increases, so does the importance of infection control. Preventing the spread of organisms which are resistant and therefore hard to treat is obviously desirable. Less obvious, but equally desirable, is control of infection by organisms which are still susceptible; every infection not prevented requires treatment, and every treatment adds to the selective pressure towards resistance.

Infection control in hospitals

4.2 In some respects, hospitals achieve the level of infection control for which they are willing or able to pay. Money can buy infection control in various ways, some of which are considered in the next few paragraphs. Standards of hospital infection control management in England and Wales were recently defined by the "Cooke Report"[45]; looking ahead, that Report said, "Antibiotic-resistant bacteria will almost certainly be an increasing problem [for hospital infection control] in the future".

Infection control teams

4.3 According to the Cooke Report (ch. 2), every acute hospital should have an infection control team.[46] The team should consist of an infection control doctor (normally a consultant medical microbiologist) and one or more infection control nurses. Non-acute hospitals should be covered, under contract, by a team from a neighbouring acute hospital. Every hospital should also be covered by a multidisciplinary Hospital Infection Control Committee.

4.4 A recognised qualification for infection control doctors has been established (DipHIC). As for nurses, the Infection Control Nurses Association (ICNA)[47] told us, "The minimum recommended training requirement for infection control nurses is a post-basic diploma-level course in infection control and previous management experience...Most NHS trusts comply with this; however some private hospitals do not" (Q 201).

4.5 The AMM reckon that each infection control nurse in the United Kingdom covers 400 acute beds (p 6). According to the ICNA (Q 201), the figure is 700; they drew our attention to US research suggesting that hospital-acquired infection could be reduced by 30 per cent by reducing the number of beds per specialist nurse to 250,[48] though they admitted that this was not quite comparing like with like. More nurses would mean a more "proactive" service, and more surveillance. The Cooke Report offers different numbers again (one nurse to 477 acute beds in 1993), but makes the same point: an understaffed infection control team can do "little more than respond to acute problems".

4.6 The ICNA claim that an infection control team is much more effective when it has resources, in terms of clerical staff and information technology. "Not all infection control nurses have access to IT; there is no doubt that this helps us in our work. None of us, or very very few, have access to a full-time secretary or a data clerk" (Q 201; on IT, cp Q 225; on support staff, cp Q 232).

---

45 *Hospital Infection Control—Guidance on the control of infection in hospitals, prepared by the Hospital Infection Working Group of the Department of Health and PHLS* (published with HSG(95)10, March 1995; see DH p 348). The Department has recently commissioned detailed clinical guidelines (QQ 755, 806–810).

46 For an account of the work of the infection control team at King's College Hospital, see Appendix 5. The experience of King's College Hospital is cited in several places in this Chapter by way of example; this is simply because that is the hospital which Sub-Committee I visited during their enquiry, and should not be taken to imply any singular praise or blame.

47 The points made by the ICNA in relation to MRSA are supported by the evidence of the Royal College of Nursing (p 451).

48 250 is the maximum permitted by the US Joint Committee for Accreditation of Healthcare Organisations, which accredits hospitals to the satisfaction of insurers.

Contracting for infection control

4.7 According to the ICNA (p 121), "The majority of infection control teams...do not have formal contracting arrangements with their purchasers". Where the contract does include the infection control team, it is often incorporated into the contract for diagnostic microbiology; according to the ICNA, "There can be virtually no resourcing within the trust for infection control because it all goes on diagnostic microbiology" (Q 232). However purchasers are currently placing less emphasis on throughput (see paragraph 4.13 below), and more on clinical outcomes (Q 232); high standards of infection control, of course, impede the former but improve the latter. The NHS Priorities and Planning Guidance (PPG) for 1997–98 requires directors of public health to ensure that adequate provision is made for infection control; "the easiest way to do this is through formal contracting arrangements".

4.8 According to Dr Mayon-White (Q 172), contracting for the infection control team is less important than contracting for high standards of infection control. The ICNA would like to see auditing against minimum standards, such as those of the King's Fund Organisational Audit, built into the contracting process (Q 232). According to Dr Graham Winyard, Deputy Chief Medical Officer and Medical Director of the NHS, the "key driver" of standards is the desire for excellence, not contractual provisions—though a contract can provide an "entrée", e.g. a seat for the Health Authority's Consultant in Communicable Disease Control (CCDC) on the Infection Control Committee (Q 805).

Hygiene

4.9 Advances in basic hygiene, both in hospitals and in the community, were reducing mortality steadily long before the discovery of antibiotics; but it is commonly believed that standards in this area are slipping, perhaps partly through over-reliance on anti-infective drugs. Poor hygiene has been definitely implicated in some outbreaks of hospital infection, and the ICNA are especially concerned about cleaning (QQ 201–9, p 124). A recent ICNA survey of hygiene in United Kingdom hospitals revealed shortcomings which the ICNA's Chairman found "quite surprising": e.g. cleaning cloths and mops going unwashed from day to day. The position has been complicated by the contracting-out of hospital cleaning services. This means that cleaners are not responsible to the ward sister, and instilling high standards and pride in the job is more difficult. High cleaning standards and training requirements may be written into the contract; but "because of cost this is often cut". The ICNA observe that there is no United Kingdom standard for hospital cleaning (p 130).

4.10 The ICNA say, "adequate and appropriate handwashing is well recognised as the single most important measure in infection control" (p 124, Q 221).[49] The AMM are also concerned about handwashing; they blame high patient turnover, and "poor provision of readily accessible hand basins", for failures in this area (p 8).

4.11 Dr Mayon-White blames falling standards of hygiene partly on penny-pinching by contractors, and partly on the loss of experienced middle managers from the NHS (Q 171). The AMM blame the pressure of high bed occupancy (p 8; see below).

Isolation

4.12 Isolation of patients is an expensive but effective form of infection control. It can take various forms: an isolation hospital, an isolation ward or "cohort nursing" within a hospital, an isolation room or side-room attached to a ward, or simply placing infected patients' beds in a corner or at the end of a row. The ICNA told us, "Most of us...have lost our isolation wards in the last five or six years...because they were no longer cost-effective to run...and now it is too late to get them

[49] The ICNA drew our attention to the particular problem of soap (Q 221). Purchase of soap is usually the responsibility of the cleaning contractor; some contractors buy cheap substandard soap. With repeated use of such soap, nurses may acquire chronic skin lesions on their hands, which render them vulnerable to chronic colonisation with MRSA. This poses no special threat to their own health; but of course it carries a risk to their patients, and sometimes means that the staff concerned must spend long periods off work. For a more sceptical treatment of hand-washing, see van Saene *et al*, p 558.

back again" (Q 219; cp Ulmanis p 528).[50] Where single rooms exist, they are sometimes carpeted—which is of no help in controlling dust-borne infections such as MRSA. Cohort nursing involves dedicating a nursing team to the affected patients; this "is becoming increasingly difficult in view of the widespread reductions in permanently employed staff, significant alterations to the nursing skill mix and an increased reliance on agency staff" (p 124).

Overcrowding and "hot-bedding"

4.13 For some years, the NHS has had a policy of maximum occupancy of beds. The ICNA report that some doctors and managers consider standard infection control measures to be "more disruptive than effective" (p 123). Maximum occupancy militates against isolation, against hygiene and cleaning, and against ward closure - "often the most effective means of control" (ICNA p 124, cp AMM p 8). It encourages hospitals to place beds too close together, which has been known to increase the chances of infection since the days of Florence Nightingale (QQ 39, 196). It also gives rise to "hot-bedding", whereby patients move frequently around the hospital as beds become free[51], potentially spreading infections as they go (AMM p 8). The shortage of beds is most acute in winter (Q 222).

4.14 While supporting the principle of efficiency, the AMM commented, "We are beginning to lose the flexibility to operate a workable infection control policy" (Q 39). They admit, "Action on resistance now is a difficult political matter since it requires diverting resources from other priorities in the short term...for what is an uncertain gain...in the future...More resources put into hospital cleaning might result in longer waiting times for treatment" (p 12).

4.15 It is of course inevitable that patients will be moved around within the hospital, and being moved is often in the best interests of the patient. The ICNA conceded, "That can be very effective bed management" (Q 223). The Minister for Public Health conceded that "Faster throughput increases risk"; but, she insisted, it is not incompatible with good practice. The message that hospital-acquired infection has an impact on both budgets and availability of beds is getting through to hospital managers. However, she admitted that "The level of control...is as good as the weakest link" (QQ 772–5).

Agency staff

4.16 A concomitant of general staff shortages and the pressure created by high bed occupancy is the increasing use of agency nurses. Agency staff are "sometimes poorly versed in infection control technique" and may be unfamiliar with local procedures (AMM p 8); and, in moving frequently from one place of work to another, they may act as carriers of infection (Q 210).

Screening

4.17 The ICNA told us that there has been a "significant rise" in screening of patients for MRSA (p 125), but that some hospitals do not currently screen at all (Q 222). However new guidelines for MRSA, currently under discussion, will recommend more rigorous screening for patients entering higher-risk units.[52] Screening takes time and costs money[53]; current techniques take 2–3 days. The ICNA say that a new molecular test takes only one day, but costs £25 per test, which "may prove prohibitive" (p 125).

4.18 According to the ICNA, there is "no expert consensus" on screening hospital staff for MRSA. However they have anecdotal evidence of staff losing jobs, or being turned down for jobs,

---

[50] Some dedicated isolation units still exist, mainly in major centres, and act as a focus of high standards of cross-infection control. Of the 1,000 beds at King's College Hospital, 63 are isolated; this, we gathered, is not enough.

[51] For example, at King's College Hospital, an 18–bed liver transplant ward saw 51 changes of bed occupant in four days.

[52] Cp van Saene *et al*, p 559.

[53] For example, at King's College Hospital, 15,000 tests are carried out each year, costing about £40,000 for consumables, £25,000 for staff and £55,000 in indirect costs. King's admits 42,000 patients per year; universal screening was once tried, but turned out not to be cost-effective.

through screening positive for MRSA, which, they observe, is not classified as an industrial disease (p 125). They also have unpublished evidence of the disruption and distress experienced by staff screened positive for MRSA (p 127).

Training

4.19 One of the roles of the infection control team is training and education. The ICNA perceive a cultural change in the United Kingdom at large, whereby good basic hygiene is no longer habitual (Q 230). Education for infection control can be delivered in various ways:

— induction courses for new hospital staff, including medical staff (Q 230). Domestic staff are in even greater need of induction, due to high turnover and lack of basic knowledge (p 126);

— in-service training: "The release...of clinical [and ancillary] staff for training is very difficult and we are getting fewer people attending educational sessions" (Q 201);

— education of patients and the public (Q 227).

As already mentioned, it is especially difficult to ensure training of agency nurses and contract cleaners. Mrs Gill Stephens, Assistant Chief Nursing Officer, insisted, "The policies are there"; but she admitted, "There are areas where improvements can be made...certain recent research has demonstrated that" (Q 773).

Infection control in the community

4.20 According to the ICNA, "Very little has been done in the community in the way of infection control" (Q 213). Some community NHS Trusts have begun to set up infection control teams, and some Consultants in Communicable Disease Control (CCDCs) at district health authority level have begun to look at the public health implications of community infection control. However most have not; and there are no national guidelines analogous to the Cooke Report for hospitals. This is of increasing importance as more health services are delivered in non-hospital settings, e.g. GPs performing minor surgery. The ICNA conclude, "Changes and developments in health care organisation and delivery have established the need for a dedicated 'community' infection control nurse role...The problems associated with the control and management of multi-resistant organisms in the community setting make it imperative that community infection control service requirements are examined and adequate provisions are made to provide an effective service" (p 121; cp AMM Q 22).

4.21 In the case of certain organisms such as MRSA, it may be argued that community infection control is not important because healthy people are not at risk. The ICNA reply that the more healthy people are colonised, the more MRSA will be carried back into hospitals to infect the vulnerable; the AMM referred to this as the "revolving door".

4.22 The ICNA gave us examples of best and worst practice (QQ 215–6). In one health authority area, with "a CCDC with vision", the infection control team have trained in MRSA control one senior member of staff from each nursing home and residential home. As a result, MRSA-positive patients do not block hospital beds while awaiting discharge into a home prepared to have them; and general standards of infection control in such homes have risen, so "We do not get the big outbreaks now". In another area, there is no community infection control nurse or public health nurse, and infection control is not part of the community trust's contract. In consequence, the infection control nurses in the local hospitals receive requests for help with community infection control, which they cannot give.

4.23 Dr Mayon-White told us that, at least in Oxfordshire where he works as a CCDC, the importance of community infection control in respect of MRSA is now well understood. He cited two reasons for this (p 107). The first was a major outbreak of MRSA around Kettering in 1991–92, involving a new strain of MRSA (type 16) which did not depend on the constant selective pressure of hospital antibiotics. The strain established itself in the community, especially in community hospitals and nursing homes, from which it was repeatedly reintroduced into Kettering hospital, and into other hospitals in the region. Control involved not only screening and isolation in the hospital, but also the establishment of a community infection control nursing service. The other cause was a sensational BBC television programme (*Panorama*) in 1996, which dramatically raised public and professional awareness of MRSA in the community: "A good thing to have come out of this scare is that the role of the community infection control team is well established in the 79 per cent of health districts [in Oxfordshire] with community infection control nurses".

4.24 For the NHS Executive, Dr Winyard acknowledged that infection control in the community is "an area of weakness" (Q 811). The Department of Health has just reviewed the role of the CCDC, and the NHS Executive is taking "active steps" to remedy certain shortcomings which emerged in some areas, notably in "proactive work" such as surveillance, policy development, research and education (p 371, Q 801). Once the current review of the Public Health (Control of Disease) Act 1984 is complete (see below), the Chief Medical Officer agreed that it might be helpful to produce a national standard for infection control management in the community, along the lines of the Cooke Report for hospitals (Q 817). The Department added, "Not every district currently has community ICN cover, but the numbers are steadily increasing. The salaries of these staff have now been excluded from the definition of health authority costs which are subject to management cost reductions in 1998/99; this should encourage more health authorities to employ them" (p 372).

4.25 The approach of nursing and residential homes to MRSA has been particularly problematical. The level of training of staff is typically low; and, as noted above, homes have tried to block admission of people carrying MRSA. The ICNA see behind this a fear of litigation and high insurance premiums (Q 231); they comment, "If nursing homes continue to refuse MRSA, they are going to run out of patients!" The Department of Health issued reassuring guidance to nursing and residential homes in 1996. The ICNA recommend that all such homes should be assessed for basic hygiene, and that staff should receive training from community infection control teams; they admit that this would be expensive (p 127).

Power to enforce treatment

4.26 If someone at large in the community carries an infection which threatens public health, such as TB, and is unable or unwilling to submit voluntarily to treatment, the public interest may demand that treatment be enforced. The Public Health (Control of Disease) Act 1984, which was largely a consolidation, gives power to a magistrate to order medical examination (ss. 35–6), and removal to and detention in hospital (ss. 37–8). Dr Mayon-White drew our attention to several shortcomings of these provisions: they give no power to enforce treatment; they place the initiative with local authorities, which used to run infectious disease hospitals but no longer do so; they assume that the best place for an infected person is hospital; they are cumbersome; and they raise questions of ethics and human rights. "They should be replaced by powers that are more sensitive to human rights, recognise the benefits of treatment, and are held by health authorities...Powers that enabled supervised treatment and care at home would be more humane and helpful..." (p 109, cp Q 185).

Surveillance

4.27 Like prudent use of antimicrobials, infection control is supported by surveillance. The PHLS told us, "The surveillance information is integral to the advice we give to infection control teams [about MRSA] on a regular basis" (p 43). We consider surveillance in detail in chapter 5.

4.28 The Department of Health and PHLS have set up the Nosocomial[54] Infection National Surveillance Scheme (NINSS), "to produce consistent, anonymised data on hospital-acquired infection to enable hospitals to compare their infection rates with others and review the efficacy of

[54] Hospital-acquired.

their infection control practices" (p 349, QQ 786–7). The Scheme so far covers bacteraemia and surgical site infection, and involves 150 acute hospitals in England; it is intended to bring in other infections and the remaining acute hospitals, to extend it to long-stay hospitals, and to set up a similar scheme in Scotland.

Infection control in prisons

4.29 Infection control in prisons in England and Wales is the responsibility of the Health Care Service for Prisoners (formerly the Prison Medical Service), which is part of the Prison Service, not the local health authority or the NHS. The situation is similar in Scotland and Northern Ireland. Dr Mayon-White finds this a problem. He calls, not necessarily for a unified service, but for "a common standard, preferably using common resources, so that it does not really matter where the infection is, it is managed as a corporate effort" (Q 152). A joint working group of the Home Office and the Department of Health is in fact currently exploring options for better integration of prison medical services with the NHS; it is expected to report to Ministers later this year.

Costs and benefits

4.30 The Cooke Report attempted to quantify the costs of hospital-acquired infections. United Kingdom data are limited, but a study in 1988 found additional costs to the hospital of between £400 and £3,200 per patient. Most of the cost arose from extra days in hospital; Dr Mary Cooke, Senior Medical Officer and principal author of the report, pointed out to us (Q 774) that this not only increases cost but also reduces patient through-put. There are also, of course, costs to the patient and to the wider community.

4.31 Individual outbreaks of hospital infection have been costed. The Cooke Report mentions several, including the Kettering outbreak of MRSA mentioned above which cost the hospital £400,000 (see Box 7). Outbreaks may have consequences beyond the direct costs: e.g. staff absences, adverse publicity, failure to meet targets due to ward closures, increased stays and general disruption. The ICNA observe, "It is difficult to justify the costs incurred from an intervention where the successful outcome measure is an event not occurring"[55]; they too cite direct costs of particular outbreaks of MRSA, including one in Madrid which involved 900 patients and cost £700,000, and they stress the wide range of headings under which costs, tangible and intangible, can arise (p 122). Dr Davey gives further examples (p 148).

4.32 Outbreaks may lead to complaints and litigation. According to the ICNA (Q 212), there has been a "tremendous increase" in complaints arising from hospital-acquired infection, and managers are becoming more aware of the implications for risk management.

4.33 Numbers can also be put on the risk to patients and the public. About one in ten patients in acute hospitals at any one time has an infection acquired after admission, according to the Cooke Report[56]; according to the AMM, the average risk to an individual patient is between 5 and 10 per cent (p 7). The risk varies according to the situation: in an intensive care unit it may be as high as one in two. Hospital-acquired infection in the United Kingdom is significant as a primary or contributory cause of death (Cooke Report 1.5).

4.34 Finally, the Cooke Report offers some indications of what effective infection control in hospitals can achieve. "We believe it is possible that currently about 30 per cent of hospital acquired infection could be prevented..." In the USA it has been calculated that a mere 6 per cent reduction pays back the cost of a three-person infection control team. A major study of 300 US hospitals over five years in the 1970s found that, while infection in hospitals with no control programmes rose by 18 per cent, rates in hospitals with control programmes including surveillance and feedback fell by 32 per cent.

---

55 Cp Greenwood p 410.

56 A survey by the Hospital Infection Society in 1994 found 9 per cent prevalence (p 421).

Box 7

COST OF MRSA OUTBREAK IN KETTERING 1991–92

Isolation wards	£303,600
Microbiology	£ 43,000
Drugs	£ 17,100
Cleaning	£ 25,600
Replacement of mattresses and pillows	£ 6,800
Community nurses	£ 7,500
	£403,600

The figure does not include the costs associated with increased length of stay, additional prescribing costs, the cost arising from absence of infected staff on sick leave or the costs of litigation.

Source: Cooke Report

A national MRSA strategy?

4.35 MRSA poses one of the biggest challenges to infection control. It is common, it moves easily between hospital and community settings, and in many United Kingdom hospitals it is now regarded as endemic. Professor Percival put it at the top of his list of problem organisms in hospitals (Q 103); and Dr Mayon-White put it top of the list of community-acquired infections (Q 149A). MRSA is treatable; but many consider that it is only a matter of time before untreatable strains emerge. That time can probably be lengthened by keeping MRSA in check. The Department of Health approved guidelines on the control of MRSA in hospitals in 1990; the BSAC, ICNA and Hospital Infection Society are currently revising them (pp 42, 349).

4.36 Dr Mayon-White calls for a national MRSA strategy (p 108, Q 168). He points out that MRSA is a marker of cross-infection generally. Therefore a strategy to control MRSA would bear down on other infections as well. He also observes that, whatever the cost of such a strategy, it would be very small compared with the cost of dealing with more outbreaks like the one in Kettering.

4.37 The Minister for Public Health spoke confidently about MRSA (Q 753). Whereas many countries now accepted MRSA as a fact of hospital life, this need not be so here; rates of resistance were relatively low[57], and the United Kingdom had "excellent clinical guidelines"[58] and surveillance which was "the best in the world". She acknowledged, however, that a "much more proactive approach" was called for, from Government and others, in order to avoid passing a "legacy" of resistance to the next generation.

[57] 8 per cent in 1990–95, compared with 30 per cent in France and 60 per cent in Japan—though differences in denominators vitiate this comparison to some extent.

[58] Currently being revised.

CHAPTER 5 SURVEILLANCE

5.1 As noted above, both prudent use of antimicrobials and infection control are informed by surveillance. Surveillance provides the information on which to base policies, and by which to assess their effectiveness. Surveillance is not cost-free; it costs money to gather and transmit information, and it costs money to collect and analyse it. Witnesses have proposed various ways to improve surveillance in the United Kingdom, of disease in general and resistance in particular, both by getting new information, and by adding value to information already available.

Duty to report

5.2 At present, in the United Kingdom, certain clinical conditions are notifiable under the Public Health (Control of Disease) Act 1984 and the Public Health (Infectious Diseases) Regulations 1988. Our witnesses point to various shortcomings of this regime.

5.3 First, there is no requirement to report resistance as such; all current reporting is voluntary. Dr Mayon-White observes that voluntary informal reporting "strains slightly the rules of medical confidentiality" (Q 177). The PHLS would like mandatory reporting, not of every resistance—"That would be far too broad and you would be overwhelmed with data" (Q 91)—but of certain key resistances either known elsewhere but not in the United Kingdom, or unknown but anticipated (Q 92). They offered a list of eight resistances; Dr Mayon-White proposed a list of just four (Q 195). See Box 8.

5.4 Secondly (AMM p 4), notifiable diseases are required to be reported to the "proper officer" appointed by the local authority; in practice this is usually the CCDC of the health authority. There is no requirement to report to PHLS. Thirdly, the regulations refer to diseases according to a very antiquated classification. In Dr Mayon-White's view, they ought to be brought in line with modern microbiology, and refer to diseases by their causative organism (Q 177). Finally, one of the notifiable diseases is "food-poisoning". As Dr Mayon-White explained, "The food poisoning statistics are a ragbag of conditions", embracing everything from *E. coli* to indigestion (Q 183).

5.5 The Department of Health informed us, "The Government is currently reviewing the provisions of the Public Health (Control of Disease) Act 1984 (and the regulations made under it) with the intention of bringing forward new legislation when Parliamentary time allows. Proposals for the new legislation will be set out in a discussion document which the Government expects to publish in the Spring. One of the provisions expected to feature in the new legislation is a requirement on laboratories to notify certain specified test results. This would be in recognition of the role laboratory testing now plays in the diagnosis of disease. It would also complement the existing system of notification of actual or suspected cases of certain diseases undertaken by registered medical practitioners. The definitive list of results to be reported would be determined in consultation with experts once the legislation has completed its passage through Parliament, but the Department will consider the inclusion of test results which can indicate some causes of hospital-acquired infection or resistance to (certain forms of) antibiotics. These are likely to include, for instance, test results indicating MRSA infection..." (letter 14.1.98, cp Q 777).

5.6 Dr Christopher Bartlett of PHLS, Director of the Communicable Disease Surveillance Centre, recommended that mandatory reporting of certain resistances be backed up by "an untoward event reporting system, in which any unusual or unexpected resistance marker in any micro-organism is reported. The advantage of this is that you can identify new antimicrobial resistance events at an early stage and implement investigations to try and sort out the determinants. Untoward event reporting has been shown to be very effective in disease surveillance" (Q 95).

Scotland and Northern Ireland

5.7 The PHLS is an agency of the Department of Health, and operates only in England and Wales. Scotland has microbiological laboratories, which report on a voluntary basis to the Scottish Centre for Infection and Environmental Health (SCIEH) of the NHS in Scotland; the SCIEH is "broadly analogous" to the PHLS Communicable Disease Surveillance Centre. PHLS-type services in Northern Ireland are provided by the Northern Ireland Public Health Laboratory in Belfast.

Box 8

MANDATORY REPORTING

Notifiable diseases under the Public Health (Control of Disease) Act 1984, s.10

* Cholera
* Plague
Relapsing fever
* Smallpox
Typhus

Also required to be notified under the 1984 Act, s.11

Food poisoning

Required to be notified under the Public Health (Infectious Diseases) Regulations 1988 (S.I.1988 No. 1546)

Acute encephalitis	Ophthalmia neonatorum
Acute poliomyelitis	Paratyphoid fever
Anthrax	* Rabies
Diphtheria	Rubella
Dysentery (amoebic or bacillary)	Scarlet fever
* Leprosy	Tetanua
Leptospirosis	Tuberculosis
* Malaria	Typhoid fever
Measles	* Viral haemorrhagic fever (including Dengue fever, Ebola virus and Lassa fever)
Meningitis	Viral hepatitis
Meningococcal septicaemia (without meningitis)	Whooping cough
Mumps	* Yellow fever

Procedure for notification

Notification under the Act and Regulations is to be made by a doctor to the "proper officer of the local authority" (normally the CCDC), and by him to the District Health Authority. The proper officer must report cases of the diseases marked *, and "any serious outbreak of any disease", to the Chief Medical Officer immediately; and must make weekly and quarterly returns of all notifiable diseases (except leprosy) to the Registrar General.

Resistances proposed to be notifiable

PHLS list (Q 92)

Organism	*Antimicrobial*
Staphylococcus aureus	Vancomycin (i.e. VRSA)
Neisseria meningitidis	Penicillin
Enterobacteriaceae (not Proteus)	Carbapenems
Acinetobacter	All β-lactams
Streptococcus pyogenes	Vancomycin
Streptococcus pneumoniae	Penicillin
Mycobacterium tuberculosis	Isoniazid and rifampicin - (i.e. MDR-TB)

Dr Mayon-White's list (Q 195)

MRSA
MDR-TB
VRE
Resistant pneumococci

Surveillance of TB and HIV/AIDS is integrated across the United Kingdom.

5.8 Dr Alasdair MacGowan, Chairman of the Working Party on Antimicrobial Resistance Surveillance of the British Society for Antimicrobial Chemotherapy (BSAC), told us, "There is a problem, in terms of integration of the various national parts of the United Kingdom, as to what we should be doing" (Q 97). Professor Brian Duerden, Deputy Director of PHLS, agreed: "We do need to improve the links with Scotland and Northern Ireland to get the national picture".

5.9 The Chief Medical Officer for England and Wales considers liaison to be good, but sees scope for improvement, e.g. in compatibility of definitions and data-collection (Q 818). The Scottish Office say, "There is evidence that reporting may be more comprehensive in Scotland" than in England and Wales[59]; a system for electronic laboratory reporting, "fully compatible" with the PHLS system, is being established in Scotland as recommended in the Pennington Report; and a recent review has recommended retaining separate Scottish reference laboratories for Salmonella, Campylobacter, *E. coli* 0157, MRSA and meningococci, rather than merging these functions with PHLS, on ground of both clinical and cost effectiveness (p 565). The Chief Medical Officer for Northern Ireland tells us that DHSS (NI) are currently working on setting up a Regional Communicable Disease Epidemiology Unit, with a view *inter alia* to "strengthening links with PHLS" (p 546).

Information technology

5.10 Surveillance is a prime target for applications of information technology, for both analysis and transmission of data; and many of our witnesses call for investment in this area (e.g. AMM Q 47, Mayon-White Q 177). The Chief Medical Officer agreed; he noted the importance of confidentiality of patient-specific data (Q 777).

Linking and feedback: the ICARE model

5.11 Value can be added to surveillance data by using information technology to link them with other data. Resistance data can be linked with records of antimicrobial usage; with clinical data from doctors submitting specimens for analysis (AMM p 5); and with clinical outcome data, to test the correlation between *in vitro* and *in vivo* (WHO Q 138; Davey p 156, Q 276). SmithKline Beecham are enthusiastic about the capacity of information from this "triangle" (usage, clinical outcome and resistance) to effect "the transformation of antibiotic use" (p 106).

5.12 Value can also be added by feeding surveillance data, with analysis and comparisons, back to those who provided it. According to the BSAC, "The PHLS at present does not regularly return analysis of the sensitivity data it collects on a routine basis to those who provide it" (p 79). The Minister for Public Health said that the PHLS is committed "in principle" to improving the situation (Q 776).

5.13 At CDC in the USA we learned about the US National Nosocomial Infection Surveillance (NNIS) system, and about Project ICARE (Intensive Care Antibiotic Resistance Epidemiology): see Box 9. We were most impressed by ICARE, and wondered how the concept might be transplanted to the United Kingdom. One way forward might be for a group of United Kingdom hospitals to ask to participate in ICARE itself; alternatively, a free-standing United Kingdom project might be supported from the NHS R&D Budget. Dr Mary Cooke, for the Department of Health (Q 786), pointed out that UK NINSS (see above, paragraph 4.28) is less developed than US NNIS, but said that incorporating prescribing information would make it more useful.

---

59 Though see the evidence of the Scottish Microbiology Association (p 470) and Dr Brian Watt (p 542).

Box 9

LINKING AND FEEDBACK IN THE USA

National Nosocomial Infection Surveillance (NNIS)

NNIS began in 1970, as a voluntary system to collect demographic and resistance data from certain wards in participating hospitals. It now involves 250 hospitals, all of 100 beds or more; it is still expanding, and becoming more representative of the generality of US hospitals. NNIS is confidential; CDC returns to each hospital its own results, in relation to the overall distribution.

Project ICARE

ICARE takes NNIS data and adds information about antibiotic usage. It currently involves 40 hospitals, each of which receives a nominal $3-4000 to support data collection; it covers 13 "bug-drug" combinations, chosen for their clinical importance. Like NNIS, ICARE is confidential; CDC returns to each hospital its own results, in relation to the overall distribution. In feeding back results to each hospital, the ICARE team at CDC try to identify interventions which can bring down rates of resistance. "One size doesn't fit all": two hospitals may have equally high levels of MRSA; in one case the cause may turn out to be overuse of cephalosporins, in the other proximity to a nursing home with poor infection control. Dr John McGowan, Professor of Infectious Diseases at Emory University, commented that, as a means of tackling resistance, ICARE has the advantage, over general guidelines, of being highly specific and taking full account of local circumstances, including constraints on resources. One limiting factor for ICARE, admitted by CDC, is the usage data; if pharmacy information exists at all, it is often set up to inform billing rather than to analyse usage. Another, pointed out by Dr McGowan, is the absence of community surveillance, which for some bug-drug combinations would be crucial.

Resources for the PHLS

5.14 The PHLS is roughly half funded by payments from the NHS and other "customers", with the balance of its budget provided by the Department of Health. The departmental contribution has been falling, and is projected to fall further:

1995–96	£52.1m (actual)
1996–97	£51.8m (actual)
1997–98	£51.9m (forecast)
1998–99	£50.9m (estimate)
1999–2000	£50.8m (estimate)
2000–2001	£50.8m (estimate)

The Minister for Public Health acknowledged that the PHLS is "an indispensable resource in protecting the public", and that the NHS must be "competent and adequately resourced" to deal with the problems of resistance; and she acknowledged the need for improved surveillance. However, she gave no indication that the Department will find more money for the PHLS (QQ 768, 779).

Crisis in clinical academic microbiology

5.15 In microbiology as in other medical specialties, clinical research is led by the clinical academic staff who combine a medical school appointment with an NHS contract. However, clinical academic posts in microbiology are currently being lost: we have heard that chairs are vacant at St Thomas' Hospital, the Royal London Hospital and King's College Hospital in London, and in Sheffield and Liverpool. The Chief Medical Officer acknowledged this problem, and is anxious to resolve it (Q 814); he pointed to the paradox that this shortage of specialists has arisen at a time of great scientific excitement for the discipline. Glaxo Wellcome identify a decline in the capacity of UK universities to conduct research and produce well-trained graduates in microbiology; this, they say, is why most of their antibacterial research is done in Italy (p 408). SmithKline Beecham likewise identify a "technology gap" and a "lack of trained people" (p 485).

5.16 SmithKline Beecham blame underfunding of the discipline "for many years". The AMM blame the Research Assessment Exercise (RAE), "which has laid greater value on the more fundamental aspects of research than those of a more practical and immediately applicable nature" (AMM p 376; cp Amyes p 544). They point out that, if funds are forthcoming for the applied research into the epidemiology and control of resistant organisms which many of our witnesses say is needed, they will be of limited use without "the very staff with the capability to lead such research and who have the credibility to ensure the implementation of any changes in practice".

5.17 We ourselves expressed concern about the state of clinical academic medicine generally, in our report *Medical Research and the NHS Reforms* in 1995 (3rd Report 1994–95, HL Paper 12). The Committee of Vice-Chancellors and Principals (CVCP) responded by setting up an independent Task Force, chaired by Sir Rex Richards, whose report *Clinical Academic Careers* was published in July 1997. We met Sir Rex to discuss his report in December 1997, as recorded in our 3rd Report of this Session (HL Paper 47). The Task Force found that medicine generally came poorly out of the RAE; they blamed the conflicting demands of teaching, research administration and clinical service, coupled with disparity of reward between clinical academics and NHS staff (3rd Report 1997–98, QQ 5–6). The CVCP has not yet responded to the Richards Report; but the NHS Executive and the Higher Education Funding Council for England (HEFCE) have already taken steps to improve liaison in connection with the RAE. In particular, as announced in June 1997 in a letter to Vice-Chancellors and others (3rd Report 1997–98, para. 8), they have set up a task group on how the RAE should treat health services research, and another on the implications for the RAE of the links between teaching, research and patient care.

A national strategy for surveillance

5.18 Professor Finch says, "At present there is no national systematic monitoring arrangement prospectively studying trends in resistance, that might provide robust data on which to make firm judgements [e.g. of the impact of OTC antibiotics]. Current data is selective in terms of sampling and is rarely denominator controlled" (p 189). The ICNA say, "There is currently no standardised national data collection system in operation in the United Kingdom which allows for comparison over time and between centres" (p 126). The AMM swell the chorus of disapproval: "The PHLS network of 48 laboratories and some NHS and university-run laboratories do collect bacterial strains of interest on a voluntary basis to send to central PHLS reference facilities or report to CDSC. Overall this has been a rather haphazard process and needs to be done systematically" (p 5, cp Q 5).[60] They go on, "Systematic collection of epidemiological data on resistance should be initiated immediately...The costs to the NHS are likely to be modest compared with many other actions" (p 14).

5.19 Cost is an issue. The AMM told us, "Most United Kingdom laboratories are not resourced to perform surveillance". According to the BSAC, "Much of the data published in medical journals derives from pharmaceutically sponsored studies [see ABPI p 177, and Box 11 below]...Although the pharmaceutical industry in conjunction with private companies, NHS and university laboratories has put considerable effort into producing good quality surveillance data so far, this has not resulted in an ongoing surveillance programme. The Government, the NHS R&D Programme and charities have not funded large-scale surveillance schemes" (p 79).

5.20 The Royal College of Pathologists define the need in terms of institutions (p 456). "We commend the apparently outmoded concept of well-found diagnostic laboratories alongside

[60] Cp also Amyes and Young, pp 374 and 376.

appropriate clinical facilities; these should be strategically sited in selected hospitals, adequately staffed...and funded...able to carry out appropriate surveillance...with results nationally and internationally co-ordinated...ready to define problems when and where they arise; and able to make persuasive applications for appropriate research funding..."

5.21 The PHLS are not defensive of the *status quo*. Dr Bartlett would like to see "support for the development of surveillance systems within an overall national surveillance strategy. At least there needs to be developed a consensus beyond the PHLS, working with colleagues in the NHS and academia, including clinicians and public health colleagues also" (Q 107).

5.22 Work on a strategy for resistance surveillance is in fact in hand. "The BSAC has recently set up a Working Party on Resistance Surveillance. It has proposed a multi-level approach to surveillance in the United Kingdom. Discussions have started with the PHLS as to how surveillance in the United Kingdom can be improved by a collaborative arrangement. In addition the BSAC is actively seeking partnerships with the pharmaceutical industry[61] and the Wellcome Trust, and has a proactive approach to implementing its concepts of surveillance during 1998 and beyond" (BSAC p 76). Details of the BSAC's proposals are given in their written evidence (p 80). The ABPI support them, and call on the Government to resource them (p 178). The Minister for Public Health said, "We support a strategic approach to this", but was unable to make any commitment as to resources (Q 778).

[61] Including Zeneca and SmithKline Beecham.

CHAPTER 6 NEW DRUG DEVELOPMENT

6.1 Another way round the problem of resistance is by using new drugs. This approach depends on the willingness of industry to invest in developing new products in this area; their success in doing so; and the ability to pay for any new patent medicines which emerge.

How hard is industry trying?

6.2 Professor Reeves of the AMM is under the impression that the pharmaceutical industry are not currently investing much in antimicrobials, because the chances of commercial return are small (Q 28). Several other witnesses told the same story (e.g. Chopra p 402).

6.3 The ABPI (p 175; QQ 314–320) tell a different tale. They acknowledge that the 1980s saw little investment in new antimicrobials. However this changed around 1990, partly because of the rise in resistance (market pull) and partly because of the "explosion of information" from bacterial genetics[62], coupled with technological improvements in drug testing (science push). "Most of the major pharmaceutical companies have invested heavily in the last five years or so in the antibacterial area", and antimicrobials are now the third largest therapeutic class in R&D, accounting for 20 per cent of pre-clinical research projects and 9 per cent of clinical development projects. It is more than 20 years since the emergence of the last major new class of antibiotics; but industry is now using genetics to look for new drug targets and modes of action, including modes of action which would either not give rise to resistance[63], or even possibly reverse it. However, new antiviral and anti-parasitic drugs are "lagging behind" antibacterials—with the exception of drugs against HIV. Three British pharmaceutical majors told us their own stories: see Box 10.

6.4 The Chief Medical Officer expressed satisfaction with the industry's efforts (Q 791): "The fact that there are not lots of new drugs coming out does not mean to say there is not a lot of work going on in this area and a great deal of investment". Professor Finch said, "[The pharmaceutical industry] have done a terrific job up till now, and maybe the new genomics is going to open up new approaches". But he warned, "We cannot always rely on [them] to come up with new agents" (Q 386).

Licensing: fast-tracking and "orphan drug" designation

6.5 The ABPI called for accelerated licensing procedures, subject to the necessary safeguards, for "new antibiotics that are acting by completely novel mechanisms of action and are active against resistant organisms" (Q 325; cp SKBp 484). The AMM make the same recommendation (Q 60); and the Chief Medical Officer is in favour of speeding up the process (Q 792). Professor Finch told us that the United Kingdom Medicines Control Agency's procedure is now very fast, and capable of responding to an application within 3–4 months. The system can be made to work even faster, and has done so for certain HIV treatments. There is also scope for compassionate use in advance of licensing. The EU Medicines Evaluation Agency takes rather longer (QQ 377–380).

6.6 If the prospective market for a new drug is not sufficiently large or wealthy to justify the cost of development, the drug is known as an "orphan". Professor Finch was unable to envisage many situations where a drug effective against a resistant infection would require orphan status rather than the normal licensing regime (Q 381). However the USA has a programme of incentives for orphan drugs, including accelerated approval and extended patent protection, and the EU is

---

62 See the evidence of the Centre for Applied Microbiology and Research (CAMR) (p 395), which also usefully surveys the leading edge of completely novel approaches to antimicrobial resistance. Novel approaches are also the subject of the evidence of Professors Brian Henderson and Michael Wilson of the Cellular Microbiology Group, Eastman Dental Institute, University College London (p 413), and are noted by the Society for General Microbiology (p 493). On bacteriophage in particular, see the evidence of Dr J Soothill (p 510). On alternative approaches involving complementary medicine, see the evidence of the Research Council for Complementary Medicine (p 447) and J Hoare (p 420). See also Appendix 6, paragraphs 49–50.

63 This "disease-based" approach is described by Glaxo Wellcome (p 406). Professor Ian Chopra, Director of a new Antimicrobial Research Centre at Leeds University, specifically seeking to promote academic–industry collaboration in discovery of antibacterial agents, warns (p 402) that there are "no reports yet even of lead molecules".

Box 10

UK PHARMACEUTICAL INDUSTRY
EXAMPLES OF INVESTMENT IN ANTI-INFECTIVES

Glaxo Wellcome (p 405)

Since 1996, anti-infectives have been one of Glaxo Wellcome's priority areas for drug discovery, with increased investment, particularly in bacterial genomics, which in their view will "fundamentally swing the pendulum back" in favour of anti-infectives.

In 1994 Glaxo Wellcome launched "Action tb", a programme for collaborative research worth £2m p.a. for five years.

Glaxo Wellcome are major contributors to the Edward Jenner Institute for Vaccines Research (see Chapter 8).

Glaxo Wellcome have agents under development against penicillin- and cephalosporin-resistant pneumococcus and staphylococcus; resistant Gram-positive pathogens and TB; and azole-resistant fungal infections.

SmithKline Beecham (SKB) (p 473)

SKB hail the genomics "revolution": but they point also to developments in chemistry (combinatorial chemistry, and biotechnology) which have vastly increased the range of chemicals available for pharmaceutical applications; and to developments in screening, enabling the new chemicals to be tested faster for effects on the new targets identified by genomics.

SKB themselves claim to have "led the pharmaceutical industry" in investment in genome sequencing; and now have a joint venture with Glaxo Wellcome to sequence bacterial genomes. They have recently given their own antibacterial research special status and dedicated resources, under the tag "Manhattan Micro".

Despite all this effort, SKB warn of a "vulnerability window between 2000 and 2007, in which multi-resistant organisms will increase in clinical importance without parallel progress in the introduction of new antibiotic classes".

Zeneca Pharmaceuticals (p 544)

Zeneca has a "significant investment" in anti-infective discovery programmes, based on genomics, but does not expect results for "many years".

consulting on a similar scheme. The ABPI support it (Q 327); SmithKline Beecham, in particular, recommend it as a way to encourage development of agents against tropical parasitic diseases (p 485); the AMM call for a United Kingdom scheme (Q 60), and Professors D A Mitchison (p 432) and A R M Coates (p 470) of St George's Hospital call for a scheme in respect of TB.

CHAPTER 7 VACCINES

7.1 In principle, any infectious disease may be combatted by vaccination, which stimulates the immune system to fight off infections which would otherwise take hold. This offers an alternative to treatment of established infections with antibiotics. Vaccination, which began in England in the late 1700s, has been one of the great medical successes of the 20th century, at least in those countries which can afford it; in the United Kingdom, for instance, vaccination has all but eliminated diphtheria, tetanus and measles, and reduced TB, mumps, Rubella (German measles) and whooping cough. The new "Hib" vaccine is highly effective against *Haemophilus influenzae* type B, formerly one of the chief causes of meningitis (Q 138). Most spectacularly, vaccination has eradicated smallpox worldwide[64], and has almost eradicated polio.

7.2 Dr Geoffrey Schild and his colleagues from the National Institute for Biological Standards and Control (NIBSC), which works with the Department of Health, PHLS and the Centre for Applied Microbiology and Research (CAMR) to evaluate vaccines for the United Kingdom, told us of the prospects for further vaccines (p 316). Prospects over the long term are good: advances in gene sequencing, molecular biology and immunology, and the production of monoclonal antibodies, are opening up new possibilities.[65] SmithKline Beecham, who have around a quarter of the world market for vaccines, agree: there is at the moment "an explosion of activity in vaccine R&D" (p 482).

HIV

7.3 Dr Schild said of HIV, "We know an enormous amount about the organism itself, but we still have no effective design for a vaccine. There are however a number of candidate vaccines under investigation" (Q 720). Dr Pillay of PHLS told us, "Progress has been very slow because we do not fully understand the nature of the immune response against HIV" (Q 590). SmithKline Beecham tell the same story, and do not expect success "in the immediate future" (p 483). The ABPI are collectively optimistic: "A vaccine for HIV infection is thought to be only a few years from marketing, assuming that remaining clinical trials are successful" (p 176).

Meningococcus

7.4 Most meningococcal infection in the United Kingdom is due to *Neisseria meningitidis* bacteria of sero-group B (two-thirds of cases) or C (one-third). A vaccine against groups A and C, suitable for people exposed to infection but not for children under two, is already available; and more effective vaccines against group C may be in use by 2000. Group B, however, presents a greater scientific challenge, and an effective vaccine may be 5–10 years off or even more (Q 720).

TB

7.5 The familiar BCG vaccine against TB, given to many British schoolchildren[66] and other people at high risk, "does not give very satisfactory protection against adult forms of the disease" (Q 721). Research is going on into alternatives, and the recent sequencing of the TB genome will "help considerably"; but a licence application may be 10–15 years away, particularly since clinical trials in TB take unusually long (Q 721), and because "the nature of protective immunity is not well understood" (SKB p 482).

---

64 For a survey of the whole subject, see *Vaccines and their future role in public health*, Parliamentary Office of Science and Technology (POST), July 1995. See in particular 3.2 and 5.2 on the risks of side-effects and adverse reactions from vaccination, which are of current concern but are not dealt with in our report.

65 Surveyed in Chapter 4 of the POST report.

66 Current practice varies from district to district.

Streptococcus pneumoniae (pneumococcus)

7.6 *Streptococcus pneumoniae* causes pneumonia, meningitis and otitis media. Several vaccines are already available, but these are not suitable for children under two and are currently given only to older people at high risk; work is in hand on more effective ones. Vaccination could reduce the problem presented by penicillin-resistant pneumococcus (Klugman p 427), which is particularly menacing in poor countries where nothing more sophisticated than penicillin is affordable (Q 144). According to SmithKline Beecham (p 483), "Vaccines suitable for infants are now in advanced stages of development...it is expected that the new generation of vaccines will become available within the next five years".

Hospital infections

7.7 There are no licensed vaccines against the common hospital infections, though some research is taking place.[67] Dr Corbel of NIBSC explained the difficulties: because of the large number of pathogens involved, most of which are found naturally in the body or the environment, universal comprehensive vaccination would be impossible. Pathogens must be targeted; he nominated Staphylococcus and Streptococcus. Patients must also be targeted; long-stay patients, and those awaiting elective surgery, might be vaccinated, but for acute patients vaccination would probably take effect too late (Q 731).

Barriers and bottlenecks

7.8 According to Dr Schild, "The United Kingdom is in an excellent position to take an international lead in vaccine development" (Q 719). "We have a very comfortable way of working with industry, which does not create conflicts of interest..." (Q 727). However Dr Corbel drew attention to two areas where there may be room for improvement. First, where research is conducted in the public sector, producing enough vaccine of adequate quality for use in clinical trials can be difficult; "The private sector is probably better set up for it" (Q 727). Secondly, the system of regulation for clinical trials makes no distinction between large-scale commercial trials and small-scale academic trials; "There might be greater co-ordination between the regulatory agencies...to make the small-scale trial simpler than it is at the moment" (Q 728).

7.9 SmithKline Beecham take a broader view (p 484): "The predicted breakthroughs in new vaccine development will not fulfil their promise if further public and political awareness of the health benefits and the cost-effectiveness of vaccination are not forthcoming. Present and future vaccines will need to be used more widely throughout the world to realise their full potential." Likewise the Royal Society (p 469): "Perhaps the question should now be asked whether the degree of risk that is deemed to be acceptable should be re-examined, and safety-testing regimes simplified in order to allow [vaccine] products to reach the market faster".

Surveillance for antigenic variation

7.10 Vaccines do not encounter resistance in the same way as therapeutic agents; but they may run up against the phenomenon of antigenic variation. An antigen is a component of an organism which evokes an immune response. Some of these responses are protective against subsequent infections. In some organisms, antigenic variation produces a rapid succession of sub-types; for instance, influenza is so variable that a new vaccine is designed every few years. In others, e.g. the pneumococcus or the common cold, numerous sub-types co-exist, making design of a comprehensive vaccine difficult or impossible (Q 751). But the possibility also exists that an apparently effective vaccine may generate selective pressure in favour of precisely those antigenic variants which will break through it, and may even encourage variation which would not otherwise take place.

7.11 Dr Schild told us that scientists are not yet sure whether this is happening or not. As we write, whooping cough is said to be breaking through vaccination in the Netherlands; but antigenic

[67] See for example SKB p 483.

variation is not the only possible explanation (Q 740). He said, "We need increasing surveillance for the possibility of the emergence of variants that may grow through vaccine-induced immunity, because of the long lead time in vaccine development" (Q 741). Such surveillance is another task for the PHLS.

7.12 International surveillance of influenza is already well established, under the aegis of the WHO; Dr Schild said, "The WHO influenza network is an example of international collaboration which time and time again has shown its value" (Q 748). Studies of protein structure may one day permit the design of an unbeatable 'flu vaccine; but for now, "We depend entirely on surveillance" (Q 752).

Research

7.13 Vaccine research is well organised and resourced around the world, but the NIBSC tell us that much more needs to be done. "There are areas where serious deficiencies in basic scientific knowledge (e.g. in some aspects of immunology, microbial genetics, epidemiology and pathogenesis) are limiting the rate of progress in extending and improving the control of infectious disease by vaccination". Work is also needed on formulation and delivery of vaccines, to reduce the complexity and cost of vaccination programmes.

7.14 United Kingdom vaccine research of a fundamental kind has received a significant boost with the establishment last year of the Edward Jenner Institute for Vaccines Research at Compton in Berkshire. The Institute will accommodate around 30 researchers, plus around 20 students and visiting scientists. Set-up costs have been found by Glaxo Wellcome, who will have first option on licensing of any products arising from research at the Institute; running costs will be shared between Glaxo Wellcome, the MRC, the BBSRC and the Department of Health.

7.15 According to the NIBSC, the existence of antibiotics has skewed vaccine research away from diseases amenable to antimicrobial treatment. With the rise of resistance to antibiotics, priorities in vaccine research require to be re-assessed. In the long run, they suggest, prevention is better than cure: vaccination is more cost-effective over time than the continual race to develop new drugs faster than the bugs can adapt to resist them.

CHAPTER 8 ANTIVIRAL DRUGS

8.1 Many people—though, on the strength of our evidence, not enough—know that some infections (e.g. salmonella, pneumonia, meningitis) are caused by bacteria, others (e.g. common cold, influenza, AIDS) by the simpler organisms called viruses. It is possible to vaccinate against some viral diseases; but until recently, most could not be treated (exceptions included herpes simplex, herpes zoster and influenza), so the question of resistance did not arise. However, since resources were poured into AIDS research in the 1980s, enormous progress has been made in understanding and treating viral infection; some new antiviral drugs are on the market, and more are undergoing clinical trials (Q 588). Like bacteria, viruses are adept at developing resistance to drugs.

8.2 Viruses are different from bacteria in some important respects. They cannot reproduce, unless they are inside a "host cell". They have no plasmids by which to transfer DNA among themselves; so, when resistance to an antiviral arises, it does so through mutation within the viral genome followed by the selective pressure of the drug. Viruses replicate very fast, giving frequent opportunities for resistant mutants to be generated. Different viruses have different "error rates" in the process of replication; HIV has such a high error rate that the viral population within any infected individual is very heterogeneous, and very likely to contain at least a few viral particles resistant to any single drug (Q 582). For more detail, see the evidence of Dr Deenan Pillay (p 278), Head of the new PHLS Antiviral Susceptibility Reference Laboratory in Birmingham.

8.3 In some cases, says Dr Pillay, the mutation which makes a virus resistant also disables it by comparison with the "wild type"; so, whereas in the presence of the drug the resistant type thrives, in its absence the resistant type is at a disadvantage. Therefore, in such cases, where a virus is transmitted to a person not previously infected and therefore not previously treated with drugs, the strain which establishes itself is the wild type, not the resistant type (QQ 586, 591; cp SKB p 478). However, "It is now becoming clear that some mutations associated with drug resistance do not actually cause resistance, but rather compensate for the loss of fitness consequent on the resistance mutation, thus generating a virus which can compete with wild type. The risk of transmission and spread of drug resistant viruses is therefore a real one, and requires close monitoring" (Pillay p 279). SmithKline Beecham tell the same story (p 479): there is no significant transmission of resistant viruses, but this "may reflect the relative infancy of anti-viral therapy".

Prudent use of antivirals

8.4 "A good antiviral agent almost by definition will generate resistance" (Q 602). As Dr Pillay explained, it is therefore necessary to use antivirals in such a way as to suppress the viral population as much as possible. He is chairing a BSAC working party, which is working on evidence-based protocols and diagnostic criteria for using antivirals; and he called for an expansion of clinical virology in hospitals (Q 611). Against HIV, as in the case of TB, giving drugs in combination is proving effective against the emergence of resistance (Q 613).[68]

8.5 Acyclovir, an antiviral against herpes simplex type one (cold sores), is already available over-the-counter in the United Kingdom for topical application.[69] Dr Pillay reported that this has so far given rise to very little resistance (Q 611).[70] However he expressed some general concern[71]: "There is no doubt that there is the potential, with the increasing amount of drugs around in the population...that may change the virus in ways we are currently unaware of" (Q 599). He called for thorough surveillance and research before more antivirals are considered for licensing

---

68 According to SmithKline Beecham, "The duration of therapy has been too short to draw any definitive conclusions on the propensity of the virus to become resistant to all three agents" (p 479).

69 Acyclovir can also be given systemically, eg in herpes simplex encephalitis; this preparation is not available OTC.

70 The rate of resistance is consistently low in the immunocompetent, but more frequent in the immunocompromised (SKB p 478).

71 Cp Greenwood p 411.

for sale OTC, and for special caution if antivirals emerge for common and highly transmissible viruses such as the common cold (Q 616).

Surveillance

8.6 As Dr Pillay explained to us (Q 594), surveillance of viral resistance is in its infancy. The PHLS Antiviral Susceptibility Reference Unit in Birmingham, of which he is the Head, was set up in 1996. It is the only service of its kind in the world, based at one of the few laboratories capable of conducting the necessary tests (Q 609). A start has been made on surveillance of herpes simplex, using a network of sentinel laboratories and targeting immuno-compromised patients; with regard to other viruses, "we are in a state of development". As noted above, methods, definitions and breakpoints for susceptibility testing of antibiotics are still a matter of debate; for antivirals, none at all have yet been validated or agreed (Q 594).

8.7 CDC in the USA, and a European network based in Holland, are working to develop surveillance of resistance in HIV (Q 595). Dr Pillay said, "The more there is an international effort in this, the better" (Q 604).

Research

8.8 According to Dr Pillay (QQ 623–632), "Antiviral research and research into basic mechanisms of viruses are going on apace, funded by the MRC, the Wellcome Trust and all the cancer charities". The NHS R&D Budget has also been forthcoming. However, the MRC has terminated its directed programme for HIV, and "it is extremely difficult to get HIV funding now through the MRC"; and HIV research is not supported by the Wellcome Trust or the major cancer charities. Dr Pillay also has difficulty raising funds for targeted research in support of surveillance; the funding bodies expect such work to be paid for by industry.

CHAPTER 9 INTERNATIONAL

9.1 Infection is no respecter of nationality or of national frontiers. Many witnesses have warned us that, although in the United Kingdom prudent use, infection control and surveillance are established to high standards, these efforts are constantly being undermined by the arrival of infections from other lands where standards are lower. A frequently-cited example is the introduction and explosive spread of penicillin-resistant pneumococci in Iceland in the early 1990s: rates rose from under one per cent in 1988 to 20–25 per cent in 1993. Subsequent studies of the genetics of the strain showed that it almost certainly came from Spain, where it was common and the usage of oral antibiotics is high (AMM p 12, PHLS p 49).

9.2 The AMM call for more action on an international scale (p 12, QQ 58–60). They call on the Government to take a lead in Europe to "raise the profile" of the resistance problem, to "create a common pool of information" on resistance and on antimicrobial usage, and to control resistant infection. "A serious attempt should be made to control resistance within Europe since it would be difficult to target developing countries before its own house were in order". Then bilaterally and through global agencies, the Government should do what it can for the wider world—though, the AMM admits, "The problems of controlling antibacterial usage in developing countries are almost insuperable".

World Health Organization

9.3 The actions of the World Health Organization (WHO) in this field are described in the evidence provided by Dr Rosamund Williams (p 91). They include assistance to developing countries to develop surveillance, using standard software (WHONET)[72] and feeding into a global "network of networks"; sponsorship of organism-specific resistance surveillance networks for gonorrhoea, TB, leprosy and malaria; education through Model Prescribing Information, a Model Formulary and national policy workshops; guidance to regulators, including Ethical Criteria on Medicinal Drug Promotion; and support for research.

9.4 The WHO Antimicrobial Resistance Monitoring programme (ARM) was set up last year, and has so far been funded largely outside the WHO budget, as is its parent, the Division of Emerging and other Communicable Diseases Surveillance and Control (EMC). The United Kingdom Department for International Development has provided a "large amount" of extrabudgetary funding for EMC, including ARM,[73] for which Dr Williams expressed thanks (Q 111). The ARM budget for 1998 and 1999 is $1.6m (about £1m) (Q 123). The WHO Executive Board has approved a Resolution[74] for the 51st World Health Assembly in May, which would draw attention to the ARM and seek to put it on a firmer financial footing (Q 117). Dr Williams indicated that the ARM would welcome secondment of experts from the United Kingdom; she suggested that this would be mutually beneficial (QQ 113–6).

9.5 Professor Petrie spoke from experience of helping to develop antibiotic policies among some of the world's poorest people (Q 669). He pointed to some of the difficulties: very little money for public health care; and often a private sector with plenty of money, eager to spend it on expensive and possibly inappropriate drugs. He added, "There is evidence in some countries that drugs are purchased for reasons which are not wholly straightforward". In this context, the WHO Essential Drugs List is important, if only as an "Aunt Sally" to begin the process of local discussion and ownership.

---

72 In Boston we met WHONET's creator, Dr Thomas O'Brien, Medical Director of Microbiology at the Brigham and Women's Hospital. See Appendix 6.

73 £2m in 1997—about half the total EMC budget—and £1m in 1998.

74 EB101.R26, 27.1.98.

Malaria

9.6 Malaria is one of the biggest global killers: it currently kills about two million people every year, and debilitates hundreds of millions more, mostly children in Africa, where the rate of transmission is very high and resources for health care are very sparse. Malaria is caused by a parasite, one of four species of Plasmodium; the parasite is injected by the bite of the Anopheles mosquito, develops in the liver, and then invades the blood to cause fever. The most dangerous type is *P. falciparum*, the cause of cerebral malaria. Between about 1950 and 1970 attempts were made through the WHO to eradicate malaria by killing the mosquitoes with DDT; this programme succeeded in some areas, but in others, notably Africa and the Far East, it failed. There followed a policy gap, during which malaria increased again. Since 1992 the world has begun again to fight back, but with a new strategy: not eradication of mosquitoes with insecticides, but treatment and prophylaxis with antimalarial drugs.

9.7 Despite climate change, there is no immediate prospect of malaria becoming endemic again in these islands (as it was in the Essex marshes and the fens in the last century) (Q 523). However malaria should be of concern to the United Kingdom for three reasons: exposure of British citizens through travel (each year the United Kingdom currently sees about 2,000 cases and an average of seven deaths); disease in Dependent Territories and the Commonwealth; and general humanitarian concern. The United Kingdom has considerable expertise in the study of malaria (MRC p 430), and a sizeable and increasing investment, notably through the Wellcome Trust (£23m in 1994–95), the MRC (which maintains a laboratory in The Gambia) and the Department for International Development.

9.8 According to Professor David Bradley and Dr David Warhurst, of the London School of Hygiene and Tropical Medicine, co-directors of the PHLS Malaria Reference Laboratory, "The spread of resistance to the common and inexpensive antimalarial drugs...is the leading cause for concern in the fight against malaria" (p 235). The leading first-line drug is chloroquine, which is cheap, easy to take and fast to act. Resistance appears to arise by a rare mutation, which may have occurred only twice, in Colombia and Vietnam; but by selection and transmission chloroquine-resistant *P. falciparum* is now encountered in all the main malaria areas (except central America, Haiti and parts of the Middle East). The other cheap first-line drug is Fansidar (pyrimethamine-sulphadoxine); resistance to this in *P. falciparum* is found at low levels even without selective pressure, and is now widespread in Africa, South America and the Far East. Newer and more expensive drugs are also encountering resistance. Resistance spreads at different rates in different places, but its rise and spread are, according to Bradley and Warhurst, "inexorable...a losing battle".

New drugs

9.9 According to Bradley and Warhurst, there is a great need for new antimalarial drugs: preferably drugs which are cheap, and chemically novel so as to reduce the chances of cross-resistance. However, "the pharmaceutical industry...is not strongly motivated to produce more medicines for impoverished people". Whereas the pharmaceutical industry looks for a market of $300m to justify the cost of developing a new drug, the world market for antimalarials is only about $100m (Warhurst Q 487), making any antimalarial an "orphan drug". According to SmithKline Beecham, industry is in fact putting "significant R&D effort" into anti-malarials, though not into other anti-parasitics of great importance to the developing world. They told us that five new anti-malarial compounds are currently under development; but each has drawbacks, and all are "likely to be much more expensive" than current drugs (p 480).

9.10 Bradley and Warhurst believe that the United Kingdom should encourage industry to develop antimalarials, by "the climate of opinion, appropriate tax relief, and support of the collaborating international agencies", perhaps by extending patent life (Q 492), and possibly in very poor countries by sharing the cost of actually buying the drugs. The WHO is already active in this area (Q 482; WHO p 93, Q 128); Professor Bradley gave us examples of two expensive new drugs which are being supplied in Africa at no cost to the users (Q 488), and mentioned a project to enable the pharmaceutical majors to collaborate on antimalarials through a "virtual company" (Q 482). He acknowledged that new drugs will in time encounter resistance as the old ones have; "Therefore it is a matter of trying to ensure a steady stream of drug availability over time" (Q 478).

9.11 One new antimalarial much talked about at the moment is artemisinin (qinghaosu). Artemisinin is derived from a Chinese medicinal plant; but its natural origins offer no special protection against resistance. Artemisinin is effective against resistant *P. falciparum* by blocking transmission of the parasite; but it is expensive, it is not suitable for prophylaxis, and in Professor Bradley's view it has been released in Africa sooner than was necessary, giving rise to a risk that resistance will develop prematurely. (See Q 479 and p 241, and MRC p 431.) SmithKline Beecham consider that the transmission-blocking action of artemisinin is promising, but "requires considerable commitment to achieve scientifically valid data with which to build drug control strategies" (p 480).

Prudent use of drugs

9.12 According to Bradley and Warhurst, "Adequate control of the drug supply is a key aspect of preventing the emergence of resistance, or at any rate of delaying it. Medicines are available in an uncontrolled way in many developing countries. High-cost unnecessary drugs are often aggressively marketed in the private sector when they are not yet needed for case management. Consequently, resistance to them may be established by the time that they are really needed. It is difficult to develop an effective licensing policy and to enforce it. United Kingdom companies are not blameless in these matters". Bradley and Warhurst call on the British Government to influence this situation in several ways: by supporting developing countries in their efforts to regulate the availability of medicines, regardless of any general preference for free trade (Bradley Q 480); by applying "appropriate pressure" to British pharmaceutical companies; and by supporting poor countries in developing drug formularies and policies.

Infection control and vaccination

9.13 With malaria as with other infections, reducing transmission of the disease reduces the need for drugs and the selective pressure towards resistance—though transmission of malaria is not person-to-person but mosquito-to-person. According to Bradley and Warhurst, there is a place for old-fashioned insecticide sprays, and for the new approach of impregnating bed-nets with insecticides (QQ 499–504; MRC p 432); and research is being carried out into genetic engineering of mosquitoes and ways to interfere with the mechanisms of pathogenicity, while work is under way to sequence the Plasmodium genome (Q 507; MRC p 430). The "best long-term hope" is a vaccine; researchers have sought for years for an effective malaria vaccine without success, but recent advances in molecular biology and increases in funding (see below) have speeded up the search (Q 506; MRC p 430).[75] Bradley and Warhurst call for increased support for research in these areas "both from and by the United Kingdom".

Surveillance

9.14 The WHO has established a general database on antimalarial resistance (p 92), and a special monitoring programme on the Burma-Thailand-Cambodia border where "the world's worst antimalarial drug resistance problem" is to be found. According to Bradley and Warhurst, "The United Kingdom needs to continue its support for surveillance programmes for drug resistance and to build overseas capacity to sustain the programmes and interpret their results". Bradley and Warhurst also call for enhanced surveillance of travellers' malaria, with which they are already involved as co-directors of the PHLS Malaria Reference Laboratory. At present, the Laboratory merely confirms the standard diagnosis. "As the genetics of resistance become clear, it is necessary to fund a reference service for detection of drug resistance genes in specimens from patients. This can also be used to provide data for endemic countries". They explained that the value of a reference genotyping service would lie "not in the management of the particular patient today, but

[75] SmithKline Beecham have a candidate vaccine which "optimistically...could be available for widespread use in 10 years' time" (p 483).

in formulating policy for the future" (Q 521). "It is essential to obtain regular data on the prophylactics used, through the international passenger survey".

Research

9.15 According to Professor Bradley, malaria research is currently enjoying a "renaissance", with plenty of scientific interest and a fair amount of funding. However, there are currently more good projects than can be supported (Q 511); and there are particular problems funding downstream, operational/health services research (Q 510). In any case, "There is a great tendency towards fashion in international funding. What is required is sustained funding for a significant period, not just the short term" (Q 505).

CHAPTER 10 RESOURCES FOR RESEARCH AND DATA-COLLECTION

10.1 We have heard from a succession of clinical academics and other scientists that little funding is available for applied research into the problems of antimicrobial resistance, or for the collection of the data necessary for systematic and effective surveillance. The position appears to be in marked contrast to the vast resources devoted, largely by the pharmaceutical companies, to basic research and drug development.

Research into different ways of using antibiotics

10.2 According to the RCGP, research funding for evaluation of different antibiotic strategies is hard to come by. The College has even taken the unusual step of providing funds itself (Q 310). Professor Finch likewise called for more research into antibiotic strategies. "We need to understand the best regimen for particular infections, not relying on those which were tested at the time of licensing in the US where the practice of medicine differs" (Q 386; cp Griffin p 548).

Research into strategies of professional and public education

10.3 Professor Peter Borriello of the PHLS, Director of the Central Public Health Laboratory, observed that, if prescribing practice does indeed affect resistance, then research is needed into what affects prescribing practice, and how best to influence it. "It is not usually the easiest thing...because you are dealing with individuals" (Q 107). According to Dr Grimshaw, this is in fact a flourishing field, with "an increasing body of international literature from rigorous studies", and a "substantive" programme of research and development funded by the NHS. "Up until now most of the evidence is North American, but the United Kingdom is rapidly catching up" (Q 672). Dr Williams of WHO likewise called for evaluation of programmes of patient/public education (QQ 119, 138).

Collection of prescribing data

10.4 The PHLS are not in a position to match patterns of prescribing with patterns of resistance (QQ 71–80, 107). Their resistance data are subject to acknowledged limitations; and they have no prescribing data at all, though some data sets exist for parts of the United Kingdom (Wales, and Tayside as described below). The PHLS have plans to begin to remedy this deficiency: in a development of TB surveillance (MYCOBNET), "it is planned to analyse treatment regimens in relation to acquired resistance"; and they are undertaking a GP research initiative by which they hope to acquire a network of sentinel practices. We were surprised to hear that they have not used PPA data for this purpose, though Professor Duerden said, "I think they should be made use of".

10.5 The Department of Health propose to collaborate with the Oxford University Unit of Health-Care Epidemiology to compare the wide regional variations in use of antibiotics noted in Chapter 2 with variations in resistance (p 344). This "will provide a useful first step in determining whether the level of community antibiotic utilisation affects the level of antibiotic resistance".

10.6 Dr Davey told us about his work at the micro-level in Tayside. With some difficulty, the Tayside Medicines Monitoring Unit have induced GPs and hospitals to use the same identifying number for each patient, so that individual records can be linked (Q 237). To improve the usefulness of the records themselves, the Infectious Diseases Unit at Ninewells Hospital has produced a stamp or sticker which prompts the doctor to write essential information in the patient's notes; but they are having difficulty exporting the concept to other units in the hospital, let alone elsewhere (p 151, Q 242). Dr Davey drew our attention to the possible implications, for use of this sort of information, of the Data Protection Bill [HL] currently before Parliament, which implements the EU Data Protection Directive (95/46/EC).

10.7 We have been told often that, whereas GPs are generally equipped to quite a high level with information systems suitable for recording and analysing prescription data, British hospitals are not (DH p 344; AMM QQ 45, 49; Davey p 150, Q 251). Dr Davey said, "Probably the single biggest fault...is that the information systems are not being designed to provide clinically useful information; they have been designed to provide information on accounting and throughput" (Q 259). Dr Winyard of the NHS Executive (Q 784) acknowledged this as "a real issue"; a few

Box 11

UK PHARMACEUTICAL INDUSTRY
EXAMPLES OF SURVEILLANCE ACTIVITIES

Glaxo Wellcome (p 407)

Glaxo Wellcome tell us that they "co-operate with local health authorities" to provide information on resistance patterns to guide prescribing. They are also "in contact with the WHO surveillance programme with the objective of both contributing to, and reacting to, knowledge of resistance emergence and spread".

SmithKline Beecham (SKB) (p 476)

According to SKB, the pharmaceutical industry has been involved in surveillance "for some time", with the aims of evaluating the medical need and commercial value of new products, and of informing appropriate use of existing ones. Industry provides funding; the work is done by clinical microbiology laboratories and research institutions; data from most such studies are published. "Overall, SKB is funding microbial susceptibility surveys in over 50 countries."

SKB claim to have been "at the forefront of a movement to address the lack of more global, longer-term studies". SKB funded the Alexander Project, to produce and publish high-quality susceptibility data for respiratory pathogens from Europe and the USA. The project began in 1992, and was extended in 1996 to countries in Asia and Africa. Other similar studies supported by industry "are now emerging".

SKB are among the companies supporting the WHO Antimicrobial Resistance Monitoring Programme. SKB contributed to the funding of WHONET (see paragraph 9.3), and support a Centre-of-Excellence Laboratory Advisory Board to help developing countries' laboratories to produce reliable surveillance data.

According to SKB, industry is "continuing to explore ways of making surveillance data available...to aid local prescribing decisions"; to aid the interpretation of the data, so as to "reduce the potential for recurrence, relapse, transmission and increase in resistance"; and to use surveillance data, prescribing data and clinical outcome data to model and predict the causes, trends and effects of resistance.

SKB acknowledge that the industry's resources put it in "a unique position" to fund data-generation. It does so "willingly, and with the goal of an increasingly evidence-based approach to antibiotic usage in mind".

Zeneca Pharmaceuticals (p 544)

"In support of our marketed anti-infectives", Zeneca recently conducted a 56-centre surveillance programme in the United Kingdom. They also have studies in Europe, and in the USA, in collaboration with CDC.

hospitals have now installed computer prescribing systems, and the Department of Health has commissioned the National Prescribing Centre to conduct a pilot study with ten of them.

Research into infection control

10.8 The preface to the Cooke Report says, "The group has been very aware of the continuing need for, and importance of, applied research into the surveillance, prevention and control of hospital-acquired infection". Professor Percival agreed (Q 108), and complained in colourful terms of the difficulty of getting grants for "pragmatic research" into, for instance, control of MRSA. Dr Mayon-White would like to see more formal trials of infection control policies; this would not be easy, but would be an improvement on "best advice and existing practice" (Q 173).

Collection of denominator data for disease surveillance

10.9 The Public Health Laboratory Service (PHLS) are the first to admit that their surveillance data have shortcomings, and one of the biggest is in the area of denominators (PHLS p 38, cp DH p 335). Generally speaking, to know that in a certain period laboratories in a certain area found X isolates of a certain organism to exhibit a certain resistance is to know little of value, beyond the clinical importance of each individual result. The laboratories can generally express X as a percentage of all isolates of that organism tested for susceptibility; the denominator is the total number of isolates tested, the number of resistant isolates being the numerator.

10.10 However this is still defective information, since laboratory isolates are only a fraction, and an unknown fraction, of all the examples of the organism at large in the area. What is worse, they are not normally a representative fraction; generally speaking, laboratories only see what doctors choose to send them (Q 77). This will tend to consist of problematical samples, including probably a higher proportion of resistant strains than is found in the general population (Q 111). It will consist largely of samples taken in hospitals (QQ 81, 383): according to the AMM, "Typically some 40 per cent of the microbiology specimens processed by a district general hospital laboratory come from the community" (p 7). It may contain multiple specimens from the same person, or specimens from persons who have infected each other (AMM p 5). It will exclude conditions such as pneumonia which do not often give rise to specimens suitable for susceptibility testing *in vitro* (i.e. in the laboratory) (Q 77). Finally, it will not be randomised for factors such as age and gender (BSAC p 78). The problem is compounded because, at present, PHLS reference laboratories only see what peripheral laboratories choose to send them. Studies funded by the pharmaceutical industry are subject to the same constraints (SKB p 477). Better denominator data can be achieved, but only with extra effort and expense.

Surveillance beyond the hospital

10.11 The PHLS admit that their data are largely confined to hospital isolates, and to isolates from invasive disease. They do not know "the wider pattern of resistance or susceptibility in the community at large, where we do not necessarily get the specimens into the laboratories. We have not conducted special surveys through the PHLS for those" (Q 71). The ICNA are particularly aware of the lack of surveillance of "community reservoirs of MRSA, especially in nursing homes" (p 126).

10.12 Dr Mayon-White similarly told us, "The study of antimicrobial resistance outside hospitals in Britain has been highly selective, typically focused on a single species or group of micro-organisms, often in one geographical area" (p 107). He advocates "the collection of comparable data on antimicrobial resistance in a number of different settings across the country" (Q 173). He told us, however, that it is difficult to find funding for such work, since it goes beyond standard service provision but falls short of research. He suggested that it might find a home in the NHS R&D programme, as "health services research" (Q 175).

10.13 In general practice, sentinel or spotter practices can be recruited, and invited to submit more specimens than would be necessary for purely clinical reasons (Q 78). Professor Finch considers that a network of such practices would provide "valuable information" (Q 384).

Research into systems of surveillance

10.14 According to Dr MacGowan of the BSAC, "We are still not very certain what the correct method of surveillance is" (Q 109). He would look to the NHS Directors of R&D to fund such work; but he fears it is not "fashionable". Likewise Dr Bartlett of PHLS calls for careful evaluation of new surveillance systems (Q 107).

A funding gap?

10.15 In short, across the range of our enquiry, there appear to be research needs, and a lack of public resources to meet them. The research in question would be highly applied, whether into better ways to use existing antibiotics, or ways to educate doctors and patients to use antibiotics more wisely, or means to prevent and control infection, or systems of disease surveillance. Some of it would amount to sheer data-collection, whether to collect the denominator data needed to put reported cases of disease in perspective, or to survey prescribing practice in order to inform the campaign for prudent use.

10.16 We put this matter to Professor Roy Anderson, a researcher in his own right in the basic but highly relevant field of population genetics, and a Governor of the Wellcome Trust. Speaking for the Trust, he acknowledged the problem: since 1992 the Trust has put around £90m into bacteriology (p 306), but only around £4.5m of that into the area of resistance. He was robustly defensive of the Trust's position: it was for the Government, not the Trust, to fund the work of public sector research establishments such as the PHLS (Q 689), and to support research to improve the operations of the NHS (Q 710). In any case, the Trust received few applications of high quality for support for work of this kind (QQ 706, 711). He acknowledged, however, that the Trust's panels of reviewers for grant applications tended to be composed of the best fundamental researchers, who might not fully appreciate the merit of more down-stream work (Q 710).

10.17 Professor Anderson indicated that the Wellcome Trust is moving to help to fill the funding gap. Scientific advances in genome sequencing (see Chapter 6) and population genetics are attracting researchers and funding to this area; and the Trust may be going to do more in future for epidemiology (QQ 686, 706). The Trust attaches importance to clinical research, and is funding research fellowships in medical microbiology (QQ 709, 713–5). Although the Trust will not support the PHLS directly, they are hoping to support university-based projects involving the PHLS in close collaboration (Q 689).

10.18 According to Professor S Amyes of Edinburgh University, whose Department of Medical Microbiology has a large research section devoted to the study of resistance, the Medical Research Council (MRC) has been notably reluctant to support bacteriology in general and resistance-related research in particular (p 544; cp Ayliffe, p 377). The MRC puts over £60m per year into immunology, infection and inflammatory disease. But most of this is basic molecular biology; expenditure specifically addressing resistance came to only £0.3m in 1995–96. The MRC say (p 429), "The current scale of research in part reflects the capacity of the academic science base to develop high quality research proposals. MRC's view is that there is potential to develop more high-quality work on resistance in the United Kingdom". In January, the MRC held an interdisciplinary workshop with the Department of Health and a number of independent experts on resistance, to explore ways in which academia might complement the efforts of industry; this recommended that clinical microbiology and antibiotic resistance should be priority areas for MRC training schemes and LINK (academic-industrial research partnership) awards.[76]

10.19 The apparent lack of high-quality proposals may be deceptive: the Royal College of Pathologists (p 455) identifies a vicious circle in operation. "The climate is such that many who would apply, decide not to do so because they are reluctant to waste their own and funders' time—and this despite funders' stated wish, at least from time to time, to support such work."

---

[76] The Biotechnology and Biological Sciences Research Council (BBSRC) also has interests in this area: see p 379.

10.20 We put the matter to the Minister for Public Health and the Chief Medical Officer, and they acknowledged the problem. The Minister said (Q 780), "The way in which research budgets are presently constructed does not necessarily mean that public health issues are given a proper opportunity to have a bid for resources". She regards this as a "fundamental problem about the structure and nature of public health research". She has already left the MRC "under absolutely no illusion" as to her view of the matter, and she intends to pursue it further. The Chief Medical Officer is similarly anxious (Q 782) that development should be supported, as well as research (e.g. resistance breakpoints, as well as basic molecular biology); he considers that this is appropriate for support from the NHS R&D budget.

CHAPTER 11 CONCLUSIONS AND RECOMMENDATIONS

11.1 **This enquiry has been an alarming experience, which leaves us convinced that resistance to antibiotics and other anti-infective agents constitutes a major threat to public health, and ought to be recognised as such more widely than it is at present.** Antimicrobial resistance is a fact of life, and the recommendations which follow will not solve the problem; but they should put the United Kingdom in a better position to face it and live with it.

Can resistance be controlled?

11.2 The evidence set out above in paragraphs 1.31–41 leads us to conclude that any antimicrobial agent must be expected to encounter resistance sooner or later. The emergence of resistance may be slow; but sometimes it is rapid, and either way it is inexorable. Resistance will take longer to emerge and spread if antimicrobial use is controlled and prudent from the start. Improving control of the use of antimicrobials can be expected to slow down the spread of resistance; and in some situations the frequency of resistance may even decline. But this must not be expected to happen in every case; and, if control is once again relaxed, reversion to high rates of resistance may be swift.

Prudent use in human medicine

11.3 The present use of antimicrobials in medicine in the United Kingdom is controlled and conservative by international standards, but on the evidence we have received (paragraphs 2.3–9) there is still plenty of room for improvement. In general practice, where most antimicrobials in human medicine are prescribed, there are wide variations in practice; many such prescriptions (witnesses offered figures ranging from 5 to 50 per cent in different settings) are unjustified on strictly clinical grounds, and where a prescription is justified the drug used is often inappropriate (and more expensive than necessary). In hospital the volume of drugs is less, and control is tighter; but even in hospital many prescriptions are made by junior doctors without proper review, and there are doubts about some aspects of present practice in relation to both treatment and prophylaxis, in particular the duration of courses.

11.4 We acknowledge the dilemma facing doctors and patients alike (paragraph 2.9), that what is prudent from the point of view of public health may be highly imprudent from the point of view of the individual patient, and *vice versa*. To use the stark example offered by the Minister for Public Health, if a child shows possible signs of meningitis, antibiotics are needed fast, and nothing must be said or done to deter the parent from seeking help or the doctor from giving it. This dilemma cannot be wished away; but we have learned that much can be done to reduce the area of uncertainty.

11.5 We commend the current trend towards local antibiotic formularies and evidence-based clinical guidelines (paragraphs 2.10–14), giving professionals agreed definitions of prudent practice in particular situations. But the issuing of documents is not enough to turn policy into practice; it must be followed through in professional education, and continuing professional development.

11.6 **We recommend that the Education Committee of the General Medical Council and the medical Royal Colleges should review the evidence presented to us** (paragraph 2.31) **that undergraduate curricula give insufficient emphasis to infectious diseases and antimicrobial therapy**. Given the consequences of poor practice for the development of resistance and therefore for public health, **the Royal Colleges should increase the attention paid to antimicrobial therapy in their programmes of postgraduate education and vocational training.**

11.7 We commend those health authorities which are devoting resources to continuing professional development of doctors in the area of prescribing. On the evidence presented to us, this is best achieved by prescribing audit and feedback (paragraph 2.34), and by educational outreach (paragraph 2.35); **we recommend that health authorities should step up their efforts in these areas**, since they are not only effective but cost-effective.

11.8 We do not recommend that GPs should be required to establish antimicrobial susceptibility before prescribing (paragraph 2.22). This, we believe, would at present be impracticable, and would overload diagnostic services which are already stretched. But improved access to microbiological testing clearly reduces uncertainty in prescribing. **We recommend that industry and the grant-giving bodies should give priority to work on rapid affordable systems for diagnosis and susceptibility testing** (paragraphs 2.16–18); **where promising developments emerge, they should be quick to move them towards the market.**

11.9 It has been put to us (paragraph 2.23) that the systems for licensing new anti-infectives could be recruited to the fight against resistance. **We recommend that the Medicines Control Agency should consider whether the drug licensing system could be used more effectively to encourage prudent use in the interest of public health.** Any change might of course involve amendment of the Medicines Act 1968.

11.10 We do not recommend further controls on the promotional activities of the pharmaceutical industry in the United Kingdom; we accept the evidence (paragraphs 2.24–25) that a system of self-regulation is in place through the ABPI. There is clear evidence that some doctors are induced to prescribe new drugs where older drugs would do; but this is a matter for the continuing professional development referred to above. **We commend the work of the WHO, through its Division of Emerging and other Communicable Diseases Surveillance and Control, to equip professionals and regulators in the developing world to respond appropriately to pharmaceutical promotions** (paragraph 9.3).

11.11 The evidence is clear (paragraphs 2.26–30) that prudent use is much harder to achieve if antimicrobials for internal use are available over the counter. **We commend the Government and the ABPI for their firm stand against over-the-counter antibiotics, and urge them not to give way.** Since this is an area of EU responsibility, and the position in several other Member States appears to be different, **we recommend that the Government should engage in active diplomacy to ensure that, should the issue be raised in the Council of Ministers, their position is understood and their allies are in place; and, in the long term, to induce those Member States which are currently more relaxed about over-the-counter antibiotics to introduce more controls.**

11.12 On the evidence presented to us (paragraphs 2.3–7), it appears that the greatest bulk of imprudent use of antimicrobials in human medicine in the United Kingdom is the prescription of antibacterials by GPs for self-limiting or viral infections and in other inappropriate situations. This encourages resistance, for example, in the pneumococcus, and might give rise to resistance in the meningococcus, which would be a disaster for public health. **The increased education for doctors which we recommend above should include education in communication skills (i.e. how to explain the reasons for refusing a prescription) and other ways to avoid prescribing on demand (e.g. delayed-action prescriptions)** (see above, paragraph 2.37).

11.13 We are disturbed by the evidence (paragraphs 2.36–39) that in many cases doctors prescribe unnecessarily under pressure from their patients, and under pressure of time. There is an urgent need for public health education in this area. We commend what is already being done; but **we urge the Government and health authorities to do more. In particular, we recommend a campaign targeted at mothers of young children**. One appropriate vehicle for such a campaign would be the popular women's magazines, with their enthusiasm for articles on health and parenting.

11.14 The message for any such campaign requires careful consideration. It would be overstating the case dangerously to say that antibiotics are bad for you; **nothing must be done to deter people from visiting their GP promptly, or from taking their medicine when necessary**. But there is evidence (paragraphs 2.40–45) that *unnecessary* antibiotics not only have public health consequences, but also increase the risk to the individual patient that any subsequent infection will involve a more resistant strain (to say nothing of the possibility of an adverse reaction to the drug itself). **The Government and the health authorities should present this evidence to the public**.

11.15 The problems of inappropriate prescribing are compounded by the failure of many patients to comply with therapy by taking their medicines as instructed (paragraphs 2.46–47); but "complete the course" is good advice only if the antibiotic is appropriate in the first place, and if the course is properly defined. **The NHS should work with the relevant professional bodies to see that courses of antibiotics are defined according to the best available current information**; wide variations in practice among different countries, as in the case of otitis media, suggest strongly that something may be wrong.

11.16 Compliance is particularly important, and particularly difficult to achieve, in cases of tuberculosis. TB services in the United Kingdom are something of which the Health Services can feel justly proud; but the recent outbreaks of MDR-TB among AIDS patients in London hospitals, and the serious problems in the USA (which cost the City of New York, for example, $175m over four years), must serve as warnings. TB services involve measures to ensure compliance[77], along with port health controls (DH p 371), surveillance and facilities for isolation; cuts in these services to save pennies today would cost this country millions of pounds tomorrow, to say nothing of the cost in human suffering. **We welcome the news that new TB guidelines from the Department of Health are to recommend more rapid diagnostic tests, and more stringent infection control, in cases of suspected MDR-TB; the Department must find the necessary resources.**

11.17 It is notoriously difficult to manage what cannot be measured; and we have heard much about the contrast between the excellent data on GP prescribing, captured by both the Prescription Pricing Authorities and GPs themselves, and the lack of data on antimicrobial use in hospitals (paragraphs 10.4–7). **We draw this to the attention of those responsible for the NHS Information Technology Strategy.** Information from the pharmacy stock-control system is not enough for these purposes; **all hospitals should install computer systems for patient-specific prescribing information at ward level.**

Prudent use in animals

11.18 Even though we made it clear from the start that use of antibiotics in animals, fish and plants was not the primary focus of this enquiry, since the Working Group of the Advisory Committee on the Microbiological Safety of Food is looking at the issue in depth, few of our medical witnesses have forborne to express concern in this area. Concern focuses on the role of the growth promoter avoparcin (which the EU has recently prohibited) in inducing resistance to vancomycin and other glycopeptides; the role of fluoroquinolones used in veterinary medicine and prophylaxis in inducing resistance to this important class of drugs in Salmonella, Campylobacter and *E. coli*; and the possibility that the growth promoter virginiamycin has already induced resistance to the new streptogramin Synercid. The evidence that we have heard (paragraphs 3.7–13) strongly suggests that **there is a continuing threat to human health from imprudent use of antibiotics in animals**.

11.19 The United Kingdom led the world in addressing the threat to human health posed by antibiotic use in farming practices with the Swann Report in 1969. Unfortunately, some of the recommendations of Swann were not acted upon and many believe that, had action been taken then, our present concerns would be much less than they are now, at least as regards the situation in the United Kingdom.

11.20 Antimicrobials are highly efficacious in animals as they are in man. The aim must be to maintain this potency. We do not go so far as some of our witnesses, who call for a ban on all growth promotion and long-term mass prophylaxis. However, on the evidence before us (paragraphs 3.20-24), we recommend that **antibiotic growth promoters such as virginiamycin,**

---

77 Including directly-observed therapy–BMA p 381.

which belong to classes of antimicrobial agent used (or proposed to be used) in man and are therefore most likely to contribute to resistance in human medicine, should be phased out, preferably by voluntary agreement between the professions and industries concerned, but by legislation if necessary.

11.21 Potent agents important to human medicine, such as the fluoroquinolones, deserve extreme economy of use in veterinary practice (paragraphs 3.15–19, 25–26). It is right for large animals and companion animals to receive such agents on an individual basis for short-term therapy; but mass-treatment of herds of pigs and flocks of poultry with such agents cannot be best practice from the point of view of human public health. **The veterinary profession must address this problem[78], by introducing rapidly a Code of Practice on when such compounds should be prescribed** (e.g. when other agents have failed) **and how** (e.g. for no longer than necessary); **we recommend self-regulation in preference to legislation.**

11.22 Many people have pointed out that, even by comparison with the human scene, surveillance of resistance patterns in animals is very limited, making analysis of the problem along the whole food chain very difficult (paragraph 3.12). **We draw this to the attention of MAFF, and of the new Food Standards Agency**, since the Minister told us that it will have surveillance as an "important function" (Q 755).

11.23 The role of farming and veterinary practice in contributing to resistance in human pathogens goes beyond the question of food, since pathogens and resistance genes originating on the farm can reach people by routes other than the food chain - for instance, via contact with companion animals. **Departmental and Agency boundaries must not be allowed to prevent the Government from getting a grip on the whole of this issue, in the interests of public health. A single multi-disciplinary Government committee to oversee all aspects of antibiotic use should now be set up, as originally recommended by the Swann Report** (paragraph 3.31).

11.24 **We draw to MAFF's attention the evidence of Dr Coles (paragraphs 3.36–41), which suggests that resistance in worms and scab pose a serious and imminent threat to the British sheep farming industry.** There is no threat to human health; but, if Dr Coles is right and if nothing is done about it, the economic consequences for farmers in the present state of the industry, and the animal welfare consequences, could be serious.

Infection control

11.25 Besides being desirable in itself, infection control is particularly important to the fight against resistance in two ways. It reduces the need for treatment and therefore the selective pressure which induces resistance in the first place; and, when resistance arises, it limits the damage by keeping the resistant organism within bounds. In respect of hospitals, the NHS is well equipped with policies for infection control; but we are not convinced that they correspond with the reality of life on the wards. We have had disturbing evidence (paragraphs 4.3–19) of infection control teams under-staffed and under-resourced; of poor standards of basic hygiene (e.g. hand-washing), exacerbated by the contracting-out of cleaning services; of inadequate facilities for isolation; of over-crowding of patients, and of "hot-bedding" with inadequate provision for infection control; and of inadequate control of agency staff, and inadequate training for all staff (including doctors, nurses and ancillary staff, and agency staff) in even the basics of hygiene.

11.26 The rise of MRSA and other hospital infections has taken place at a time when the Health Services have placed emphasis on patient throughput and economy; this may have led some managers and clinicians to see infection control as a cost and an impediment, rather than a basic component of patient care. The present Government express determination to change the ethos of the Health Services in this respect. As one practical way to do so, **purchasers and commissioning agencies should put infection control and basic hygiene where they belong, at the heart of**

[78] The evidence of the British Veterinary Association (p 393) suggests that they are already doing so.

good hospital management and practice, and should redirect resources accordingly. The evidence of the cost of hospital-acquired infection (paragraphs 4.30–34) suggests that **such a policy will pay for itself quite quickly**. In particular, **the NHS Executive should assure themselves that every NHS hospital is covered by a properly trained infection control team**, as recommended in the Cooke Report.

11.27 While we do not go so far as to recommend a national task force against MRSA, we found what the Department of Health had to say on this subject complacent (paragraphs 4.35–37). Levels of MRSA in this country are low by international standards, but they are rising. The more MRSA circulates, the more vancomycin must be used to treat it, bringing closer the prospect of VRSA which in the words of the PHLS would be "catastrophic" (p 44, Q 95). **We recommend that the NHS should set itself targets for controlling MRSA in hospitals, and publish its achievements.**

11.28 As Dr Winyard himself acknowledged (Q 811), infection control beyond the hospital is an area of particular weakness (paragraphs 4.20–25). This is especially true of nursing and residential homes, which can act as reservoirs of MRSA and other resistant organisms which are carried back into hospitals again and again. As a step towards improving the situation, we recommend that, once the current review of the Public Health (Control of Disease) Act 1984 is concluded, **the NHS should draw up national standards and guidelines for community infection control management**, along the lines of the Cooke Report for hospitals. **These should include a requirement that every district health authority should have at least one community infection control nurse**. Such an exercise might also usefully include the special factors affecting prisons (paragraph 4.29).

11.29 **We draw to the attention of those responsible for the review of the Public Health (Control of Disease) Act 1984 Dr Mayon-White's evidence** (paragraph 4.26) **as to shortcomings of the provisions for compulsory medical examination and detention in hospital, and the case for a more humane regime, and for extending the legislation to provide also for supervised treatment at home**.

Surveillance

11.30 Surveillance—the collection of microbiological data for comparison, analysis and feedback—is vital to the fight against resistance. It supports prudent prescribing, by tracking the rise of resistance, and informing local formularies and policies accordingly; and it supports infection control, by giving warning of areas of weakness. In both areas, it allows practice to be evaluated by revealing its effects on local rates of resistance and infection.

11.31 The PHLS were admirably frank with us about the shortcomings of their surveillance, especially in the area of denominator information (paragraphs 10.9–10). **We recommend that the NHS R&D Directorate should support microbiological surveillance among the population at large, with a view to improving denominator information, as a legitimate call on the NHS R&D Budget.** This is just the sort of public health research which we had in mind in 1988 when we first recommended that there should be a NHS R&D Budget.[79] **The MRC and the medical charities should also be prepared to support such work**.

11.32 **It is astonishing that the Departmental subvention for the PHLS is falling** (paragraph 5.14), **at a time when surveillance of infectious disease and particularly resistant disease has become so important. The Department of Health must reconsider these cuts.**

11.33 **We draw to the attention of those responsible for the review of the notification provisions of the Public Health (Control of Disease) Act 1984 the proposals of our witnesses** (paragraphs 5.2–6) **for reporting of diseases by causative organism, and for mandatory**

[79] *Priorities in Medical Research*, 3rd Report 1987–88, HL Paper 54.

reporting of certain resistances. Any increase in the burden of reporting placed on hospital laboratories will have resource implications which the NHS must face; and it must be matched by an improvement in the level of feedback from the PHLS.

11.34 We recommend that Health Ministers assure themselves that liaison between the PHLS and its analogues in Scotland (especially in the context of impending Devolution) and Northern Ireland is as close as possible (paragraphs 5.7–9). **In particular, Ministers should set a deadline for full compatibility of definitions and data-collection**.

11.35 **We draw to the attention of those responsible for the NHS Information Technology Strategy the scope for IT to facilitate surveillance of disease and resistance** (paragraph 5.10), particularly by speeding up exchange of compatible data locally, nationally and internationally, and by permitting links to be made between microbiological data and clinical data of prescribing and outcomes, subject to the necessary safeguards for confidentiality of patient-specific information.

11.36 We congratulate the PHLS and the NHS on the establishment of the Nosocomial Infection National Surveillance System (NINSS) (paragraphs 5.11–13). The usefulness of NINSS will be much enhanced if it can be linked with data on the use of antimicrobials. **We recommend that the NHS should examine the ICARE Project run by the US Centers for Communicable Disease Control and Prevention (CDC), and consider the possibility of setting up something similar, possibly in partnership with CDC.**

11.37 We commend the efforts of the BSAC and the PHLS to put resistance surveillance on a more strategic and comprehensive footing (paragraphs 5.18–22). **The Government must engage constructively with those involved, and find additional resources.** Surveillance depends on many microbiological laboratories in the NHS and the medical schools, as well as those which are part of the PHLS, and we have received evidence that these are generally under-staffed; **we recommend that NHS Trusts and universities should examine their priorities in this area.**

11.38 We are concerned at evidence (paragraphs 5.15–17) that clinical academic microbiology, which provides much of the expertise for surveillance, and for infectious disease medicine generally, is currently failing to attract recruits and fill senior posts. The problem is widely acknowledged; **it must be addressed by the NHS, the Higher Education Funding Councils, and the heads of medical schools**. This may be a special case of a more general problem concerning the pressures placed on clinical academic medicine by the conflicting demands of the Research Assessment Exercise and the ever-growing burdens of teaching, service provision and administration; **we have expressed concern about this before, and we do so again**.

New drug development

11.39 We congratulate the British pharmaceutical industry for renewing their efforts to find novel antimicrobials (paragraphs 6.2–4). We wish them success; but results cannot be expected in the short term. Pharmaceutical development is a very lengthy process; drugs at the R&D stage today may not be on the market for several years, during which time resistance to existing drugs could get dramatically worse. The sequencing of complete genomes, such as that of *Mycobacterium tuberculosis* which was achieved at Hinxton Hall as our enquiry drew to a close, is a great achievement, but only a first step; there are numerous other steps between a gene sequence and a new drug product, including characterisation of the gene products and the trial of many possible drug targets.

11.40 We commend the EU proposal for an "orphan drug" regime (paragraph 6.6). **The Government should respond positively, and should seek to ensure that the scheme gives the pharmaceutical industry a real incentive to work on novel treatments for problem diseases, particularly diseases of the world's poor such as malaria** where the market is at present worth relatively little but the cost in human suffering is huge.

Vaccines

11.41 As more antimicrobials lose their effectiveness, the importance of vaccines grows (see Chapter 7). What is more, like other forms of infection control, vaccines act against resistance at source, by reducing the amount of antimicrobial chemotherapy required and therefore reducing the selective pressure on bacterial populations. **We commend the establishment of the Edward Jenner Institute. The numerous agencies committed to research into effective vaccines must keep up the good work**. Vaccines effective against malaria, group B meningococcus and HIV, and more effective vaccines against the pneumococcus and TB, would be particularly valuable.

Viruses

11.42 As new antivirals reach the market (see Chapter 8), **the NHS must ensure that they are used prudently from the start, and that changes in susceptibility are monitored**. The lessons learned from 50 years of use and abuse of antibacterials must be fully applied.

11.43 **We congratulate the PHLS on establishing the world's first reference laboratory for antiviral resistance**, under Dr Deenan Pillay in Birmingham. **The PHLS must adequately resource the development of this important field.**

International

11.44 Resistant bacteria do not respect frontiers. The international trade in food of all kinds exposes British shoppers to the consequences of the misuse of antibiotics in farming practice around the world. In the era of mass travel by air, a resistant bacterium of gonorrhoea (for example) may evolve in Bangkok one day and be in Birmingham the next. Public health in the United Kingdom is therefore affected directly, for better or worse, by action or inaction in other parts of the world.

11.45 We commend the Government, and particularly the Department for International Development, for their exemplary support over recent years for the WHO Division of Emerging Diseases (paragraph 9.4). **This support should be maintained, and the United Kingdom Government's example should encourage other nations and agencies to contribute to this vital work. We endorse the resolution on this subject which is to be considered by the World Health Assembly in May; we urge the Assembly to pass it.**

11.46 The United Kingdom has had a good record of support for malaria research, and for the efforts of the WHO to help poor countries to combat this disease (paragraphs 9.6–15). **The Government and the grant-awarding bodies must maintain this record**.

Resources for research and data-collection

11.47 There is still much that needs to be done to increase understanding of the mechanisms of resistance and the action of antimicrobials and, in the clinical sphere, methods of using agents to best advantage (paragraphs 10.2–14). There are data to be collected on resistance and use (in animals and man), and how to prevent the emergence and spread of resistant pathogens (bacterial, viral, fungal and parasitic); and many educational ventures are required in order to find the most suitable approaches to control the problem.

11.48 Research in this area evidently falls between a number of stools (paragraphs 10.15–20), receiving inadequate support from the major grant-giving bodies and the NHS R&D Strategy. **The grant-awarding bodies and the NHS Executive should reconsider the important public health issues surrounding antimicrobial research, and should give such research an enhanced priority.** As in the case of surveillance, **we particularly commend this as a suitable area of activity for the NHS R&D Strategy.**

11.49 We note that both the MRC and the Wellcome Trust report a shortage of high-quality research proposals in this area. **We challenge the research community to come forward with proposals which, given the increased interest in the field which is already apparent, will fully justify support from the grant-awarding bodies.**

11.50 Although research including surveillance is imperative, it should not take the place of immediate action to improve antibiotic use and prevent the spread of infections.

Information technology

11.51 Information technology can play a major role in the fight against antimicrobial resistance, in three main areas: audit of antibiotic usage (see above, paragraphs 11.7 and 17), collection and analysis of disease surveillance data (paragraph 11.35), and linkage of the one with the other. The full benefits of IT in this area, as in others, will only be realised when every GP, every hospital ward and infection control team, and every clinical microbiology laboratory, has compatible and interconnected IT. **The NHS Executive must work towards this goal, accepting that it will involve considerable cost, and giving a strong lead from the centre to ensure compatibility.**

An epidemic in its own right

11.52 It will be apparent from the above that we take the issue of resistance to antibiotics extremely seriously. The evidence we have received is alarming enough as to the present situation, and even more so as to the prospect for the future. In the long term, science may come to the rescue, with novel antimicrobials and additional vaccines; but in the short term the world is facing what may be described as an epidemic in its own right, and the dire prospect of revisiting the pre-antibiotic era.

11.53 As things stand, the United Kingdom has much to be grateful for, and a certain amount to be proud of. Rates of resistance here are lower than in most countries, and the health care professions are doing their best to keep them so; and our contribution to the fight against resistant disease in other parts of the world is considerable. But the trend of resistance is upward, and we are not convinced that either Ministers[80], the public or the veterinary and agricultural community have fully grasped the importance of action in the short term. The health care professions may have a better grasp of the problem, but lack the resources to address it vigorously. To the extent that the problem is understood, the fact that it crosses several departmental and disciplinary boundaries is impeding action; hence our recommendation for a multidisciplinary interdepartmental committee as recommended by Swann.

11.54 We do not wish to overstate the problem, at least as it affects the United Kingdom. This country is facing nothing like the continuing tragedy of malaria in Africa. But food poisoning and hospital-acquired infection are already at levels which cause concern, and, if action is not taken now, it is quite conceivable that VRSA, or further outbreaks of MDR-TB, may arise here, with all the consequences of suffering and expense. **The Government clearly desire to develop a strategy to safeguard the effectiveness of antimicrobials; we conclude by urging them to follow this project through along the lines recommended in this report, to back it with resources, and to set themselves and the Health Services challenging targets for real improvement. Antimicrobial resistance is here to stay; but action or inaction now, not only by the Government but by everyone with a stake in public health, will have a real impact on the public health legacy which we pass on to the next generation.**

---

[80] The Chief Medical Officer has made it clear in his annual reports for 1995 and 1996, and in his evidence to us (QQ 756, 765) that he is seized of the problem. Ministers will shortly receive advice on prudent use in human medicine from a sub-committee of the Standing Medical Advisory Committee (Q 759), and on prudent use in animals from the Advisory Committee on Microbiological Safety of Food (see above, Chapter 3).

CHAPTER 12 SUMMARY OF RECOMMENDATIONS

A major threat

12.1 This enquiry has been an alarming experience, which leaves us convinced that resistance to antibiotics and other anti-infective agents constitutes a major threat to public health, and ought to be recognised as such more widely than it is at present (see above, paragraph 11.1).

Prudent use in human medicine

12.2 With a view to encouraging more prudent use of antimicrobials, health authorities should step up continuing professional development of doctors in the area of prescribing, especially by prescribing audit and feedback; by educational outreach; and, for GPs, by education in communication skills and other ways to avoid prescribing on demand (paragraphs 11.7 and 11.12).

12.3 The Government and the health authorities must do more to educate the public about the proper use of antimicrobials. In particular, we recommend a campaign targeted at mothers of young children. Nothing must be done to deter people from visiting their GP promptly, or from taking their medicine when necessary; but the evidence that *unnecessary* antibiotics not only have public health consequences, but also increase the risk to the individual patient that any subsequent infection will involve a more resistant strain, should be presented to the public (paragraphs 11.13–14).

12.4 We also recommend that—

(i) The Education Committee of the General Medical Council and the medical Royal Colleges should review the evidence that undergraduate curricula give insufficient emphasis to infectious diseases and antimicrobial therapy, and the Royal Colleges should increase the attention paid to antimicrobial therapy in their programmes of postgraduate education and vocational training (paragraph 11.6);

(ii) Industry and the grant-giving bodies should give priority to work on rapid affordable systems for diagnosis and susceptibility testing; where promising developments emerge, they should be quick to move them towards the market (paragraph 11.8);

(iii) The Medicines Control Agency should consider whether the drug licensing system could be used more effectively to encourage prudent use in the interest of public health (paragraph 11.9);

(iv) The Government and the ABPI must maintain their firm stand against over-the-counter antibiotics. The Government should engage in active diplomacy to ensure that, should the issue be raised in the EU Council of Ministers, their position is understood and their allies are in place; and, in the long term, to induce those Member States which are currently more relaxed about over-the-counter antibiotics to introduce more controls (paragraph 11.11);

(v) The NHS should work with the relevant professional bodies to see that courses of antibiotics are defined according to the best available current information (paragraph 11.15);

(vi) While the new guidelines from the Department of Health, recommending more rapid diagnostic tests and more stringent infection control in cases of suspected MDR-TB, are welcome, the Department must find the necessary resources (paragraph 11.16);

(vii) Those responsible for the NHS Information Technology Strategy should consider the contrast between the excellent data on GP prescribing, captured by both the Prescription Pricing Authorities and GPs themselves, and the lack of data on antimicrobial use in hospitals. All hospitals should install computer systems for patient-specific prescribing information at ward level (paragraph 11.17);

and we commend the work of the WHO, through its Division of Emerging and other Communicable Diseases Surveillance and Control, to equip professionals and regulators in the developing world to respond appropriately to pharmaceutical promotions (paragraph 11.10).

Prudent use in animals

12.5 There is a continuing threat to human health from imprudent use of antibiotics in animals (paragraph 11.18).

12.6 Antibiotic growth promoters such as virginiamycin, which belong to classes of antimicrobial agent used (or proposed to be used) in man and are therefore most likely to contribute to resistance in human medicine, should be phased out, preferably by voluntary agreement between the professions and industries concerned, but by legislation if necessary (paragraph 11.20).

12.7 The veterinary profession must address the problem of over-use of fluoroquinolones and other potent agents of importance to human medicine by introducing rapidly a Code of Practice on when and how such compounds should be prescribed (paragraph 11.21).

12.8 We also recommend that—

(i) MAFF and the new Food Standards Agency should consider the need to improve surveillance of resistance patterns in animals (paragraph 11.22);

(ii) Departmental and Agency boundaries must not be allowed to prevent the Government from getting a grip on the whole of the issue of resistance, in the interests of public health. A single multi-disciplinary Government committee to oversee all aspects of antibiotic use, as recommended by the Swann report, should now be established (paragraph 11.23);

(iii) MAFF should consider the evidence of Dr Coles which suggests that resistance in worms and scab pose a threat to the British sheep farming industry (paragraph 11.24).

Infection control

12.9 Purchasers and commissioning agencies for hospital services should put infection control and basic hygiene where they belong, at the heart of good hospital management and practice, and should redirect resources accordingly; such a policy will pay for itself quite quickly. The NHS Executive should assure themselves that every NHS hospital is covered by a properly trained infection control team, as recommended in the Cooke Report (paragraph 11.26).

12.10 The NHS should set itself targets for controlling MRSA in hospitals, and publish its achievements (paragraph 11.27).

12.11 The NHS should draw up national standards and guidelines for community infection control management, along the lines of the Cooke Report for hospitals. These should include a requirement that every district health authority should have at least one community infection control nurse (paragraph 11.28).

12.12 Those responsible for the review of the Public Health (Control of Disease) Act 1984 should consider Dr Mayon-White's evidence as to shortcomings of the provisions for compulsory medical examination and detention in hospital, and the case for a more humane regime, and for extending the legislation to provide also for supervised treatment at home (paragraph 11.29).

Surveillance

12.13 The Government should engage constructively with the efforts of the BSAC and the PHLS to put resistance surveillance on a more strategic and comprehensive footing, and should find additional resources. NHS Trusts and universities should examine their priorities in the resourcing of their microbiological laboratories (paragraph 11.37).

12.14 The Department of Health must reconsider the cuts in the Departmental subvention for the PHLS (paragraph 11.32).

12.15 We also recommend that—

(i) The NHS R&D Directorate should support microbiological surveillance among the population at large, with a view to improving denominator information, as a legitimate call on the NHS R&D Budget. The MRC and the medical charities should also be prepared to support such work (paragraph 11.31);

(ii) Those responsible for the review of the notification provisions of the 1984 Act should consider the proposals of our witnesses for reporting of diseases by causative organism, and for mandatory reporting of certain resistances. The NHS must face the resource implications of any increase in the burden of reporting placed on hospital laboratories; and the level of feedback from the PHLS must be correspondingly improved (paragraph 11.33);

(iii) Health Ministers should set a deadline for full compatibility of definitions and data-collection between the PHLS and its analogues in Scotland and Northern Ireland (paragraph 11.34);

(iv) Those responsible for the NHS Information Technology Strategy should consider the scope for IT to facilitate surveillance (paragraph 11.35);

(v) The NHS should examine the ICARE Project run by the US Centers for Communicable Disease Control and Prevention (CDC), and consider the possibility of setting up something similar, possibly in partnership with CDC (paragraph 11.36);

(vi) The failure of clinical academic microbiology to attract recruits and fill senior posts must be addressed by the NHS, the HEFCs and the heads of medical schools. This seems to be a special case of a more general problem concerning the pressures placed on clinical academic medicine by the conflicting demands of the Research Assessment Exercise and the ever-growing burdens of teaching, service provision and administration; we have expressed concern about this before, and we do so again (paragraph 11.38).

New drug development

12.16 The Government should respond positively to the EU proposal for an "orphan drug" regime, and should seek to ensure that the scheme gives the pharmaceutical industry a real incentive to work on novel treatments for problem diseases, particularly diseases of the world's poor such as malaria (paragraph 11.40).

Vaccines

12.17 We commend the establishment of the Edward Jenner Institute. The numerous agencies committed to research into effective vaccines must keep up the good work (paragraph 11.41).

Antiviral drugs

12.18 As new antivirals reach the market, the NHS must ensure that they are used prudently from the start, and that changes in susceptibility are monitored (paragraph 11.42). The PHLS reference laboratory for antiviral resistance must be adequately resourced (paragraph 11.43).

International

12.19 The Government's exemplary support for the WHO Division of Emerging Diseases should be maintained, and the United Kingdom Government's example should encourage other nations and agencies to contribute to this vital work. We endorse the resolution on this subject which is to be considered by the World Health Assembly in May; we hope that the Assembly will pass it. The United Kingdom's good record of support for malaria research, and for the efforts of the WHO to help poor countries to combat this disease, must be maintained by the Government and the grant-awarding bodies (paragraphs 11.45-46).

Resources for research and data-collection

12.20 Grant-awarding bodies and the NHS Executive should reconsider the important public health issues surrounding antimicrobial research and give such research an enhanced priority. This is a particularly suitable area of activity for the NHS R&D Strategy. We challenge the research community to come forward with proposals for antimicrobial research which will fully justify support from the grant-awarding bodies (paragraphs 11.48-49).

Information technology

12.21 The NHS Executive must work towards the goal of compatible and interconnected IT for every GP, every hospital ward and infection control team, and every clinical microbiology laboratory. They must accept the considerable cost involved; and they must give a strong lead from the centre to ensure compatibility (paragraph 11.51).

A national strategy

12.22 The Government should develop a strategy to safeguard the effectiveness of antimicrobials along the lines recommended in this report; they should back it with resources; and they should set themselves and the Health Services challenging targets for real improvement (paragraph 11.54).

APPENDIX 1

Members of the Sub-Committee who conducted the inquiry

Lord Dixon-Smith
Lord Gregson
Lord Jenkin of Roding
Baroness McFarlane of Llandaff*
Baroness Masham of Ilton*
Lord Perry of Walton
Baroness Platt of Writtle
Lord Porter of Luddenham
Lord Rea*
Lord Soulsby of Swaffham Prior (*Chairman*)
Lord Walton of Detchant*
Lord Winston

* *Co-opted members*

The Sub-Committee appointed as its Specialist Advisers:

Professor Harold Lambert, Emeritus Professor of Microbial Diseases, St George's Hospital, Tooting

Professor Richard Wise, Professor of Clinical Microbiology, Birmingham City Hospital

APPENDIX 2

Witnesses

The following witnesses gave evidence. Those marked * gave oral evidence.

Advisory Committee on the Microbiological Safety of Food
Professor S G B Amyes & Dr H-K Young
* Association of Medical Microbiologists
* Association of the British Pharmaceutical Industry (ABPI)
Professor G A J Ayliffe
Dr B Bannister
Dr J Bates
* Dr R Bax
Biotechnology and Biological Sciences Research Council (BBSRC)
* Professor D Bradley and Dr D Warhurst
British Association for Chemical Specialities
British Embassy, Tokyo
British Medical Association
British Pharmacological Society
British Poultry Meat Federation
* British Society for Antimicrobial Chemotherapy (BSAC)
British Veterinary Association
Centre for Applied Microbiology and Research (CAMR)
Dr P L Chiodini
Professor I Chopra
* Dr G Coles
* Dr P Davey
Dr D W Denning
Department of Health and Social Services, Northern Ireland
* Department of Health
* Professor R Finch
Glaxo Wellcome
Professor D Greenwood
Professor G E Griffin
* Dr J Grimshaw
Professor B Henderson and Professor M Wilson
Dr R L R Hill
J Hoare, Veterinary Surgeon
Hospital Infection Society
* Infection Control Nurses' Association
Infection Control Team, North Middlesex Hospital
Institute of Biology
Dr H F Kennedy and Dr J R Michie, Royal Hospital for Sick Children, Glasgow
Professor K Klugman
Mrs L H Lewy
* Dr R Mayon-White
* Dr H McGavock
Medical Research Council (MRC)
Ministry of Agriculture, Fisheries and Food
Professor D A Mitchison
Dr J Monro
Monsanto Europe
Dr P Murphy
National Anti-Vivisection Society
* National Institute for Biological Standards and Control (NIBSC)
* National Office of Animal Health (NOAH) and FEDESA
Osborne Practice, Southsea
* Professor J Petrie
Dr L J V Piddock
* Dr D Pillay

* Public Health Laboratory Service (PHLS)
Research Council for Complementary Medicine
* Royal College of General Practitioners
Royal College of Nursing
Royal College of Pathologists
Royal Pharmaceutical Society of Great Britain
Royal Society
St George's Hospital Medical School, Department of Medical Microbiology
Dr H K F van Saene *et al*
Scottish Microbiology Association
Scottish Office
* Dr N Simmons
SmithKline Beecham Pharmaceuticals
Society for General Microbiology
Soil Association
Dr J Soothill
Dr R C Spencer
Dr J Sterland
Dr E J Sweeney
Dr D Tyrrell
Dr G Ulmanis
United Kingdom Agricultural Supply Trade Association (UKASTA)
United Kingdom National Committee for Microbiology
Dr B Watt
* Wellcome Trust
* World Health Organization (WHO)
Zeneca Pharmaceuticals

APPENDIX 3

Visit to Public Health Laboratory Service Headquarters, Colindale, 22 July 1997

1. Six members of the Sub-Committee, with staff, met at the headquarters of the Public Health Laboratory Service (PHLS) in Colindale, for informal briefing on PHLS's work on infections resistant to antibiotics.

2. **Professor Brian Duerden**, Deputy Director, introduced PHLS. PHLS is funded by the Department of Health and the Welsh Office to provide microbiology and epidemiology services in England and Wales. It has two central facilities in Colindale, the Central Public Health Laboratory (CPHL—microbiology) and the Communicable Diseases Surveillance Centre (CDSC—epidemiology), and 48 Public Health Laboratories at NHS hospitals around the country. There are Reference Laboratories at CPHL, and some of the PHLs have Reference Units for particular infections. PHLS has close contact with the many NHS clinical microbiology laboratories which are not PHLs, and with the corresponding services in Scotland, Northern Ireland and the Irish Republic.

3. PHLS can track the micro-organisms causing disease and monitor their resistance to antimicrobial agents in three ways:

(i) general surveillance: all laboratories regularly report all cases of specified infections to the centre;

(ii) Reference Laboratories receive micro-organisms and data for more detailed investigations; they may in turn rely on a network of "sentinel laboratories" for specific surveillance;

(iii) special "snapshot" surveys of limited duration, organised from the centre.

4. These processes are not without problems. First, they depend on voluntary reporting; PHLS would like to see legislation for mandatory reporting. Secondly, they do not provide "denominator" data: i.e. how reported cases compare with the situation in the population at large. Thirdly, they are skewed by the tendency for most Reference Laboratories (other than the Laboratory for Enteric Pathogens: see below) to see only "interesting" cases, including cases exhibiting resistance. Fourthly, they depend on different laboratories working to standards and definitions which are both reliable and compatible. All PHLS and NHS laboratories are regularly tested with blind samples sent round by NEQAS; the British Society for Antimicrobial Chemotherapy (BSAC) currently has a group working on standard methods for the UK (with PHLS input); and the EU and the USA have a task force on co-ordinated surveillance; but the situation remains far from perfect.

5. **Dr Barry Cookson**, Director, Laboratory for Hospital Infection, CPHL, spoke about methicillin-resistant *Staphylococcus aureus* (MRSA). SA is present in the nose of one person in three (persistent in one in ten, otherwise transient), and is not usually resistant; but resistance develops rapidly, usually in the context of a hospital. SA colonises skin but usually cannot invade it unless there is a wound; if it does invade, and sepsis arises, it becomes serious. SA is spread by direct contact.

6. "We are running out of antibiotics." In the 1970s MRSA in the UK was checked, by a combination of gentamicin and better infection control; but in the 1980s MRSA developed gentamicin-resistance. In the UK MRSA can still be treated with vancomycin and a number of other antibiotics. But in some parts of the world vancomycin may be the only effective antibiotic, and low-level vancomycin-resistant MRSA has emerged in Japan.

7. MRSA prevalence varies widely between countries, regions, hospitals, and even individual wards. However two recent strains, EMRSA–15 and –16, have spread across the UK and crossed to Holland. EMRSA–16 can be virulent; it is the first strain with two super-antigens, and can cause chest infections in particular.

8. Ways to control MRSA include infection control, policies to control use of antibiotics, and other factors such as staff to patient ratios; but no system is wholly reliable. Nurses are crucial,

since they have most direct contact with patients. Any survey of MRSA in a hospital must take account of how many carriers brought it in with them. Many serious cases arise from auto-infection, e.g. in a patient already carrying MRSA who undergoes surgery and whose lesions are then invaded as they heal.

9. **Dr David Livermore**, Head, Antibiotic Reference Unit, CPHL (from 1st September 1997), described the work of the ARU: it tests "difficult" organisms for susceptibility or resistance to antibiotics, and checks surprising results from other laboratories; it monitors and researches resistant strains, and provides advice; and it supplies strains for use by NEQAS.

10. ARU is trying to move from snapshot surveys, which are resource-intensive, to continuous local monitoring. As noted above, this depends on quality assurance (QA); susceptibility-testing in the UK is much less uniform than in the USA. BSAC and PHLS are currently testing new methods, and PHLS hope to have sentinel laboratories in place by the end of 1998.

11. Dr Livermore mentioned penicillin-resistance in *Streptococcus pneumoniae* (= pneumococcus). In the UK resistance has risen to about 4 per cent. Iceland has suffered a dramatic rise, from one per cent in 1980 to 30 per cent in 1990. This is believed to have originated via travellers returning from Spain.

12. Dr Livermore also mentioned resistance to vancomycin. Because of how this antibiotic works (it binds to a substrate rather than an enzyme), resistance was thought to be impossible. However in about 1987 there emerged the vancomycin-resistant enterococcus (VRE); how this came about is a mystery. As to why, it happened while avoparcin, a related antibiotic, was being used in Europe as an animal growth-promoter. This "can't have helped"; but the human and animal strains of enterococcus concerned are not the same; and the USA has more VRE than Europe, although avoparcin is not used there. Plasmid transfer of vancomycin-resistance to MRSA is now a "substantial risk", and has been demonstrated in the laboratory on the skin of a mouse; but the low-level VRSA found in Japan is not due to gene transfer and probably arose by mutation.

13. **Dr Bernard Rowe**, Director, Laboratory for Enteric Pathogens, CPHL, regards resistance to antibiotics as "unwelcome but inevitable". He spoke about salmonella, of which there are about 2000 serotypes, causing typhoid, paratyphoid and enterocolitis, most commonly due to food poisoning.

14. Since 1989, *Salmonella typhi* has acquired resistance to chloramphenicol; the incidence is now around 30 per cent. Resistance emerged in India and Pakistan, and most cases found in the UK can be traced to infection in SE Asia.

15. There are about 30,000 cases a year of human salmonella food-poisoning in England and Wales, mostly acquired by eating UK food. As the table shows, multi-drug resistance is now most common in *S. typhimurium*, the second most prevalent serotype in humans in the UK. A particularly worrying strain is *S. typhimurium* DT104, which is multi-resistant. This is the major cause of salmonellosis in cattle, sheep, pigs and poultry; it also infects humans, and its spectrum of resistance is widening. Dr Rowe attributes this to use of antibiotics in food animals. For instance, late in 1993 enrofloxacin was licensed for veterinary use; DT104 promptly acquired resistance to the very similar human antibiotic ciprofloxacin. It should be noted that, though highly resistant, DT104 is no more virulent for humans than other salmonellae, and in most cases antibiotics are not required.

16. Dr Rowe believes that farmers are using antibiotics as a substitute for good hygiene and husbandry; in his view, the ban on use of human antibiotics as animal growth promoters, introduced after the Swann Report of 1969, should be extended to cover prophylaxis. (There is a grey area around "metaphylaxis": treatment of animals believed to be incubating disease.) He detects a recent change of heart on this issue in agribusiness.

Multi-drug resistance in Salmonella in England and Wales, 1990–96

	Per cent of salmonellosis in humans 1996	MDR per cent 1990	MDR per cent 1996
S. enteritidis	63	0.8	0.6
S. typhimurium	19	18	90
S. virchow	4	11	19
S. hadar	2	2	56

MDR = Multi-drug resistant, i.e. to four or more antibiotics

17. **Dr Patrick Wall**, Consultant Epidemiologist, CDSC, described ENTERNET, a project for international surveillance of food poisoning. ENTERNET, funded by the EU under BIOMED, involves EU member states and also Switzerland and Norway. It began as Salm-Net to monitor salmonellae, and has been extended to take in the antibiotic resistance of salmonellae and *E. coli 0157*. Participating laboratories commit themselves to acquire a minimum data set, and training in standard methods is provided by PHLS if required. Dr Wall gave striking examples of successful "detective work", identifying international outbreaks of food poisoning and tracing them to their source. Recently the food industry has become more involved with the PHLS in initiatives to improve the safety of food, and PHLS are now working with the supermarkets to develop codes of practice for food production and handling.

18. **Dr Francis Drobniewski**, Mycobacterium Reference Unit, Dulwich PHL, spoke about multi-drug resistant tuberculosis (MDR–TB—defined as resistant to isoniazid and rifampicin). TB is responsible for more deaths worldwide than any other infectious disease (3m per year). The emergence of resistance is encouraged by failure of patients to complete antibiotic courses (typically 6 months or longer), by poor prescribing, and by the physiology of certain groups of patients, particularly people with AIDS, among whom MDR–TB causes 80–90 per cent mortality. There have been two recent outbreaks of MDR–TB among people with AIDS in London hospitals (Chelsea and Westminster 1995, St Thomas' 1996); these have given rise to expensive litigation, and a major programme to build negative-pressure isolation rooms. The WHO has set up a Global Surveillance System, involving 22 reference laboratories of which the MRU is one. The MRU has been appointed the WHO European Region Co-ordinating Laboratory in recognition of its work in the field of drug resistance. There is a lot of MDR–TB in Eastern Europe; the eastward expansion of the EU is therefore a cause for concern.

19. **Dr J Watson**, Consultant Epidemiologist, CDSC, described MYCOBNET, the UK surveillance system for TB set up in 1995. Data for the whole UK is collected at PHLS CDSC. In the UK as a whole MDR–TB is rare but increasing; it is concentrated in London, among people with AIDS, among recent immigrants (50 per cent of TB patients in the UK were born overseas; screening on or after arrival is impractical), among homeless people (who are particularly prone to non-compliance) and among people who have had TB before. MDR–TB is a global problem; but, as a recent WHO review has shown, data from around the world are patchy and inconsistent.

20. **Dr Ros Stanwell-Smith**, Consultant Epidemiologist, CDSC, stressed the need not merely to "count corpses", but to improve the situation by changing behaviour. In her view, PHLS leads the world at the former but could do more of the latter. By way of example, she described how she provides surgeons with prompt and graphic feedback concerning resistant infection of surgical wounds. Hospital policies on use of antibiotics are effective only if staff can be persuaded to follow them; one good way to find out what is actually happening is to ask patients. Continuing education of medical staff is a key activity.

APPENDIX 4

Visit to Public Health Laboratory Service Headquarters, Colindale, 23 October 1997

1. Three members of the Sub-Committee, with staff, paid a second visit to PHLS at Colindale.

2. Dr David Livermore showed us the **Antibiotic Reference Unit**, where isolates referred from hospitals are tested for susceptibility or resistance. Usually only unusual or problematic isolates are referred (except for TB and salmonella); hence the selectivity of surveillance. We were shown four different kinds of test.

(i) The pathogen is cultured on an agar plate, and discs of antibacterial agent are then placed on the plate. A clear circle round the disc indicates susceptibility. This test takes two days; it is cheap (10p per disc); it is only semi-quantitative.

(ii) The pathogen is cultured on an agar plate, then the antibacterial agent is introduced on a strip marked with an ascending scale of concentration. This test is more expensive (£1.50 per strip) and no faster, but quantifies the "minimum inhibitory concentration" (MIC).

(iii) The pathogen is cultured on a series of plates containing an antibacterial agent in increasing concentrations, to identify the MIC. We saw a computer-assisted technique for reading the plates, but this still relied heavily on human hand and eye.

(iv) The pathogen is tested for the presence of genes associated with resistance, using the polymerase chain reaction (PCR). This test is more expensive than tests (i)—(iii) (£5 per test), and only slightly faster; and each test will only show the presence or absence of a single known gene. We saw simple kits in use; automated systems are under commercial development.

3. We asked about the application of digital imaging to these tests; we were told that automation in microbiology is lagging behind other laboratory disciplines.

4. Dr Barry Cookson showed us the **Laboratory of Hospital Infection**, and discussed his survey of infection control teams and MRSA in 1995. He noted that antibiotic policies are best informed by setting information about local prescribing patterns against information about local resistance patterns: paradoxically, in hospitals, microbiological information tends to be good while prescribing information tends to be poor, while in general practice the situation is reversed. He found only three hospitals where antibiotics policies were firmly based on the findings of local surveillance; and he pointed to King's College Hospital as an unusual example of success in using local infection data to negotiate for more resources for infection control. In general practice, PHLS aims to set up a network of 50 sentinel practices; but it is hard to persuade a GP to devote time and money to testing, until empirical treatment has been tried and failed.

5. Dr Cookson mentioned that, on a surgical ward, the rate of patients colonised with SA who develop infection may be one in four. He commented on the very low incidence of MRSA in the Netherlands: infection control is stringent; and, because of the low incidence, stringent control is affordable. He also commented on the British National Formulary: much good information, but presented in an "unfriendly" fashion. He noted the particular difficulty, in surveillance of MRSA, of establishing the source of infection.

6. Dr Bernard Rowe showed us the **Laboratory of Enteric Pathogens**. This is the national reference laboratory for food-borne pathogens, and is linked to other reference laboratories in Europe via ENTERNET, funded by the EU; it is also a WHO Collaborating Centre for resistant strains. The Laboratory receives 95 per cent of all human salmonellas isolated in the UK (except Scotland) and the Republic of Ireland, amounting to 30,000 isolates per year; it receives another 20,000 isolates per year of *E. coli* and other pathogens; it tests up to 300 isolates per day, and has a database going back 30 years. (Salmonella in animals is notifiable to the Central Veterinary Laboratory under the Zoonoses Regulations.)

7. Dr Rowe insisted that the problem of resistant salmonella was due to the use of antimicrobials in animal husbandry as prophylactics (treating healthy animals) or "metaphylactics" (treating healthy animals which have been exposed to disease). Resistance in salmonella does not normally threaten the individual patient, because in most cases recovery takes place without treatment; but it increases the survival and spread of salmonella in animals and therefore the overall level of human food poisoning. There was no suggestion that genuinely sick animals should not be treated; and, since the Swann Report of 1969, the use as animal growth-promoters of antibiotics used, or related to those used, in human medicine has been prohibited in the UK.

8. We heard about the case of apramycin, a veterinary antibiotic for calves. It is now known that use of apramycin gives rise to resistance to gentamicin, an important clinical antibiotic. Apparently, the industry was aware of this, but waited until it was established by published research before voluntarily withdrawing apramycin.

9. We also heard about the case of enrofloxacin, licensed by MAFF for animal use in 1993, in the face of scientific advice that it would give rise to resistance to ciprofloxacin. Since 1994, *Salmonella typhimurium DT 104* has acquired chromosomal resistance to ciprofloxacin. It was suggested that this was a case of "agency capture", and that an independent Food Standards Agency might have acted differently.

10. Dr John Watson told us about the **Communicable Disease Surveillance Centre**, of whose respiratory diseases group he is the head. CDSC has recently taken over from OPCS the receipt of statutory notifications of infectious diseases. Dr Watson explained the dual purpose of surveillance: to advise individual doctors how to treat individual cases or groups of cases; and to inform general treatment guidelines.

11. Dr Watson spoke mostly about TB. UK surveillance of TB is comprehensive, and co-ordinated since 1993 by "MYCOBNET". A detailed survey is conducted every 5 years. Compared with salmonella, TB produces fewer isolates (15,000 in 4 years, compared with 30,000 in one); and isolates seen by the reference laboratory represent a much higher proportion of all cases. (In TB 60 per cent of cases are identified microbiologically, the rest clinically or by X-ray; in salmonella only about one per cent of cases are identified at all.) In the UK, TB resistance to isoniazid is stable at 6 per cent, slightly lower than in the USA; resistance to isoniazid and rifampicin ("multi-drug resistance", MDR) is low (1–2 per cent) but clearly rising.

APPENDIX 5

Visit to King's College Hospital, 4 November 1997

Introduction

1. Seven members of the Sub-Committee, with staff, visited King's College Hospital on Denmark Hill.

2. **Professor Mark Casewell**, Professor of Medical Microbiology, introduced the hospital: a London teaching hospital, with approximately 1,000 beds including 100 high-dependency beds and 3,500 admissions per month; the UK centre for liver transplants, which carry a high risk of hospital-acquired infection and would be impossible without antibiotics; and an academic centre for the study of antibiotic-resistant organisms and hospital infection control.

3. Professor Casewell gave a general introduction to the issues surrounding resistance. The organisms of most concern at King's are MRSA[1], Klebsiella and other coliforms; VRE; and MDR–TB. Of these, VRE alone is sometimes literally untreatable; Professor Casewell described the experience, unnerving to a doctor trained in the age of antibiotics, of facing a patient with an infection where no treatment exists. He drew our attention to the medico-legal question, whether patients coming into hospital should be forewarned of the risk of contracting a resistant infection. Commenting on the theory that "the era of antibiotics is over", he remarked that, if so, this would have profound consequences for modern medical and surgical practice.

4. Professor Casewell is not convinced that resistance to vancomycin is due to use of avoparcin in animals. He pointed out that the USA does not use avoparcin but has plenty of VRE; and he referred to unpublished research suggesting that the vancomycin-resistance transposons in humans and animals are distinct. He admitted being "out on a limb" on this issue.

Medical Microbiology Laboratory

5. We visited the laboratory, and saw susceptibility/resistance testing in progress. Three years ago King's set up a bench dedicated to screening for MRSA; now 15,000 tests are carried out each year, costing about £40,000 for consumables, £25,000 for staff, and £55,000 in indirect costs.

6. Professor Casewell regards the development of an overnight test for MRSA as a top-priority research project. He described the close relationship between the medical microbiologist and the clinician as "pivotal", and a great asset to UK medicine, shared by Spain, Holland and Scandinavia, but not found in France, Germany, southern Europe, the USA or Japan, where the hospital laboratory is more like a cheaper "results-only factory".

7. At King's, 6–7 per cent of patients contract a hospital-acquired infection; 10–20 per 1,000 become colonised with MRSA; and 2–4 per 1,000 become infected with MRSA. Professor Casewell knows of no other UK hospital with such firm incidence data. He considers that such data ought to be compiled nationwide, as they are in Spain and the USA. He acknowledged the problems of inadequate IT, and reluctance to publish poor figures.

Infection Control Team

8. We met two nurses from the Infection Control Team. The full Team is unusually well-staffed: one doctor, three nurses, a secretary and an IT specialist. The nurses explained how, when notified of an infection, they inspect the ward, talk to the patient and their family, and give instructions to the nurses and other staff. To clear patients colonised with MRSA, they use Bactroban, a nasal form of mupirocin invented at King's. Decolonisation typically takes one to three weeks. When patients are discharged, a letter is written to the receiving institution or GP. Sometimes other hospitals, and even other units within King's, will not receive a patient unless they have a negative screen for MRSA. In King's catchment area, there is no infection control team in the community; this was felt to be a serious failing.

9. The nurses reckoned that factors making for poor infection control include a poor environment, low morale, inadequate staffing and excessive use of agency staff. Professor Casewell contrasted the UK approach, tailoring infection control to the circumstances of the ward

---

1 See the evidence of Dr R Hill of King's, p 417.

or patient, with the US approach of universal precautions: the UK approach seems to be more effective in practice.

10. **Dr Jim Wade**, Infection Control Doctor, explained that MRSA is endemic in King's, as in most hospitals in the South East of England, and that therefore it was necessary to a certain extent to "ride the wave". Screening and search-and-destroy methods were targeted at those patients and units most at risk. Two or three times a year it might be necessary to restrict admissions to a particular ward while an outbreak was dealt with; the extreme step of closing a ward, with all its consequences for patients and the Trust, was taken only rarely.

Surgical Ward

11. We visited an orthopaedic ward: a long room of the Nightingale type. Isolation is not practical in such a setting, so patients colonised with MRSA are moved; there was currently a colonised patient in a two-bed side ward, effectively blocking the other bed. Across the hospital, 16 patients with MRSA were currently in isolation.

12. Infection control on this ward was evidently effective: there had been no ward closure, or even an outbreak of more than two related infections, for about three years. Universal screening for MRSA had been tried, but was not found to be cost-effective, so was not currently done.

13. We asked about handwashing: at King's, nurses use a good liquid soap, without antiseptic, and this seems to be effective. We also asked about "bank" and "agency" nurses: the proportion of temporary nursing staff on a ward can range from 10 per cent to as much as 50 per cent; agency nurses pose a particular challenge to infection control, since they are not screened and may be unfamiliar with local infection control procedures.

14. Professor Casewell commented that three features of current hospital practice militate against infection control: the lack of side wards and isolation facilities (King's has 63: 22 in medicine, 5 in surgery, 19 in specialties and 17 in the private wing); the downgrading of the ward sister, who should be a senior nurse in a position to keep tight control of procedures even for temporary staff; and the acute shortage of beds in London, brought about by the Tomlinson Report, which led to "hot-bedding"—he gave examples from King's of an 18–bed liver transplant ward which saw 51 changes in bed occupants in four days, and a 12–bed ward which in the same period saw 22.

15. **Mr Matthew Porteous**, Consultant Orthopaedic Surgeon, and **Janice Allen**, Senior Ward Sister, handed in the attached note of recommendations.

Intensive Care Unit

16. We visited the Intensive Care Unit, where up to one patient in two will contract a hospital-acquired infection. In the last four years, there have been three deaths possibly attributable to MRSA after heart surgery, and one from VRE. There have also been deaths from Gram-negative organisms such as Klebsiella; these are different in that the pathogen is not acquired from the hospital environment, but is already present in the patient before becoming invasive. The ward had two isolation rooms, with both positive and negative pressure ventilation. (Positive stops bacteria from the general environment reaching the patient; negative stops bacteria from the patient getting into the hospital.) However, some highly-dependent patients cannot be safely isolated because their medical condition is unstable and requires constant attention.

17. **Dr Max Ervine**, Consultant Anaesthetist, said that the ICU tends to import MRSA from elsewhere. He drew attention to the problem of moving colonised and infected patients out to other parts of the hospital, because of the general shortage of side-wards.

MDR–TB

18. **Dr Anton Pozniak** spoke about multi-drug-resistant TB. The incidence in London is low but rising, and the cost of each patient to the NHS is very high. MDR–TB kills 46 per cent of HIV-negative sufferers, and a much higher proportion of those who already have HIV. The USA had experienced many outbreaks in 1990–92, following the dismantling of public health prevention programmes in the 1980s; he hoped that the same mistake would not be made here.

19. He mentioned the two recent outbreaks of MDR–TB in London, involving eight patients (all HIV+) at the Chelsea and Westminster, and seven patients (six HIV+) at St Thomas'. These outbreaks had been contained; but in Argentina one HIV unit had suffered an outbreak which infected 162 people and killed 146 of them. Two particular problems of such outbreaks were the

difficulty of tracing everyone who might have had contact with the infected persons, and the real hazard to medical staff.

Discussion

20. *Prescribing policies* King's has recently tightened up its antibiotic policies. One way in which such policies are implemented is through "restrictive reporting" by the laboratory, whereby the microbiologist reports in the first instance only those susceptibilities which would enable the referring doctor to treat within the policy. (E.g. if the bacterium is susceptible to antibiotics A and B, and the policy is to prefer A, only susceptibility to A is reported.) Restrictive reporting is common practice in England, but not elsewhere. Professor Casewell noted that levels of resistance tend to be lower in countries with rigorous prescribing policies (e.g. Scandinavia, the Netherlands), and higher in countries with less control (e.g. southern Europe, the USA).

21. *Prisons* TB is unusual in UK prisons. However, there was support for the suggestion that prison medical services should be more integrated with the NHS.

22. *Leg ulcers* Dr M Edmonds, a consultant physician, showed horrific pictures of the effect of MRSA on leg ulcers in diabetic patients.

23. *Research* Dr Mufti, Consultant Haematologist, said that research in this area, both health services research (e.g. into whether cohort nursing or isolation makes for better infection control) and biomedical research into alternative approaches to infection, was badly needed and under-funded, and the pharmaceutical industry could not be relied upon to make the running. It was suggested that this would be a good call on the NHS Research and Development budget.

Public education

24. It was suggested that the UK is not as good at educating the public in these matters as, for instance, the USA or Germany; and that the contribution of the media was particularly disappointing.

DEPARTMENT OF TRAUMA AND ORTHOPAEDICS, KING'S COLLEGE HOSPITAL
Antibiotic Resistant Bacteria—A Surgical Viewpoint

1. These bacteria are here to stay; the development of increasingly resistant strains seems inevitable. It may be possible to slow this process by a more meticulous antibiotic prescribing policy.

2. These bacteria—particularly methicillin resistant *Staphylococcus aureus* (MRSA)—pose an infection risk in all surgery. The consequences of such infection in Trauma and Orthopaedics are devastating as most operations in this specialty involve the insertion of foreign material (e.g. a plate for a fracture or a hip or knee replacement), infection of which usually leads to the need for removal of the metalwork and total failure of the operation. Infection of this type in the elderly carries a significant mortality.

3. Eradication of these bacteria has not worked and it seems more practical to adopt a policy of containment such as we use in this hospital. The work of the Control of Infection Team has been highly effective in implementing this policy at King's and minimising disruption of the service.

4. This policy is not universal and considerable difficulty can be experienced in inter-hospital transfers of patients who have not been screened for MRSA which can incur delays of up to a week. The adoption of an NHS-wide policy in this respect is advocated.

5. The layout of older hospitals with large open wards and few if any single rooms does not lend itself to the easy isolation of patients infected with or carrying resistant bacteria, without a significant impact on service provision.

6. Temporary staff on wards are reluctant to nurse MRSA patients as there is no provision for their sick leave if they become carriers of the bacteria.

7. Provision should be made to recognise persistent carrying of resistant bacteria by nursing and medical staff as an industrial disease.

Matthew Porteous
Consultant Orthopaedic Surgeon

Janice Allen
Senior Ward Sister

APPENDIX 6

Visit to the United States of America, 16–21 November 1997
Note by the Chairman

1. I and three other members of the Sub-Committee, one of our Specialist Advisers and our Clerk visited the USA for five days in November 1997, to meet US and international experts in the field. We did so because the USA has similar problems to the UK, but on a larger scale; many of the world's experts are there; and the US approaches to surveillance and control are different, and might, we thought, carry lessons for the UK.

2. My companions were Baroness Masham of Ilton; Lord Perry of Walton; Lord Rea; Professor Richard Wise; and Mr Andrew Makower. The travellers cannot praise too highly the many busy people, whose names appear below, who made time to prepare for our visit, to receive us on our travels, and to impart the information and ideas which this note attempts to synthesise. We also wish to place on record our gratitude for the help which we received from HE Sir Christopher Meyer KCMG, HM Ambassador to the USA, Mr Peter Marshall CMG, HM Consul General in Atlanta, Mr Jim Poston, HM Consul General in Boston, and their staffs, and in particular from Mr Roy Forey, Science and Technology Officer at the British Embassy, who accompanied us on our travels.

3. This note is in two parts. The first deals thematically with aspects of the subject on which the travellers brought home new insights and information, finishing with a list of "take-home messages". The second part is a diary.

4. The cost of the visit was just under £30,000.

POLITICAL PROFILE OF INFECTIOUS DISEASES

5. Infectious diseases, and resistance in particular, are rising up the US political scale; this can be measured by examining the budgets approved by Congress. The report by the Institute of Medicine, "Emerging Infections: Microbial threats to health in the US", published in 1992, identified resistance as a major factor in the (re-) emergence of infections; the report evidently made a deep impression, and has largely set the US agenda ever since. Other factors include concerns about biological warfare (Iraq) or terrorism (the Tokyo underground incident); and the presence in the Senate of the transplant surgeon Bill Frist.

6. Staff of OSTP revealed how the report of the Institute of Medicine led to action at the highest level. It was taken up by the National Science and Technology Council and the inter-agency Committee for International Science and Technology; and their recommendations were embodied in 1996 in a Presidential Directive (roughly equivalent to a White Paper). This established a task force on emerging infections, chaired by CDC and OSTP. The task force has set up a sub-group on resistance, to look at matters including surveillance, animal feed additives, and public and professional education. CDC has made it one of its five priorities to "expand our capacity to respond to urgent health threats", including resistant organisms; has published a strategic plan, "Addressing emerging infectious disease threats: A prevention strategy for the US"; and is organising an International Conference on Emerging Infectious Diseases in March 1998 in Atlanta.

7. Like the UK, the USA is also very concerned about food poisoning: see below.

HOSPITAL INFECTIONS

8. NIAID believes that around 2m people acquire infection in US hospitals every year, at a total cost for additional treatment of $4.5bn. More precise costs are hard to come by; but it has been calculated that, in New York City in 1995, there were 13,550 Staphylococcal infections, causing 1,400 deaths and treatment costing $435.5m.

9. Dr Levin of Emory University pointed out two obstacles to surveillance of hospital infections: outcomes may be obscured bacause the patient is already in poor shape, especially in intensive care; and hospitals may be reluctant to conduct rigorous surveillance, since every infection identified counts against them in any league table.

Vancomycin intermediate-resistant Staphylococcus aureus (VISA)

10. VISA was first reported in Japan in 1996. In 1997 two cases were reported in the USA: one in a peritoneal dialysis patient, the other in a patient infected repeatedly with MRSA. Both patients were successfully treated.

11. People at FDA told us that they had been expecting fully vancomycin-resistant *Staph aureus* (VRSA), and that VISA had come as a surprise. Dr Heyse of NIAID expressed doubt whether the VISA recently identified in the USA was a new development, or something which had existed for some time before being spotted. Dr Jarvis at CDC fears that VISA may be only an intermediate step on the way to VRSA.

12. CDC, NIH and FDA have been working with the pharmaceutical industry to look for existing drugs, possibly unexploited, which might be effective against VRSA; they have looked at 300 candidates, and shortlisted 10. FDA is standing by to grant accelerated approval. Meanwhile, hospitals are attempting to keep VRE and MRSA apart, to prevent the creation of VISA/VRSA by exchange of genetic material.

Methicillin-resistant Staphylococcus aureus (MRSA)

13. The proportion of MRSA among strains of *Staph aureus* in large US teaching hospitals rose from 8 per cent in 1986 to 40 per cent in 1992. In New York City in 1995 the proportion was 50 per cent. We heard remarkably little about it, indicating perhaps that it is now simply a fact of life in US hospitals.

14. MRSA is not notifiable in the USA.

Vancomycin-resistant enterococcus (VRE)

15. VRE is much more of a problem in US hospitals than in the UK; but Dr Levy of Tufts University pointed out that, as MRSA increases, so does the use of vancomycin, bringing VRE in its wake. The proportion of US hospital-acquired enterococci found in non-critical care units and reported as resistant to vancomycin rose from 4.9 per cent in 1993 to 9.1 per cent in 1994. In intensive care units, where vancomycin use and resistance are higher, VRE as a proportion of all E rose from 11.5 per cent to 13.6 per cent over the same period. VRE has also risen as a proportion of all US hospital infections, from 0.3 per cent in 1989 to 7.9 per cent in 1993.

16. A few States have made VRE notifiable.

GLOBAL KILLERS

Multi-drug resistant tuberculosis (MDR–TB)

17. TB is unusual among infectious diseases: the mycobacteria multiply relatively slowly, so the incubation period and the courses of treatment required are exceptionally long. These factors affect control and compliance, and therefore affect resistance. Resistance in TB first arises by spontaneous random mutation of the mycobacterium; it is then fostered by selective pressure induced by poor prescribing and non-compliance with therapy.

18. Around the world, TB is on the increase, and MDR–TB is a global problem: a recent WHO report has identified several "hot zones", mainly in Eastern Europe and South America. In the USA, total TB rose from 22,200 cases in 1985 to 26,700 cases in 1992, but has since fallen back to 21,337 cases in 1996; however in some areas (e.g. Washington DC) it is still rising, for a range of reasons. In the early '90s, the USA suffered several mini-epidemics of MDR–TB: the worst was in New York, where at its height MDR–TB accounted for 15 per cent of all TB, concentrated particularly among homeless persons, prisoners and people with HIV. MDR–TB now accounts for 2 per cent of all TB in the USA; one case in two among people aged 25–44 is associated with HIV.

19. MDR–TB carries a high mortality, and is much more difficult and expensive to treat than susceptible TB. Dr Ginsberg of NIAID told us that multi-drug resistance raises the cost per case from $200 to $200,000: most of this is accounted for by expensive drugs and long stays in hospital. From 1993 to 1996, the number and proportion of US cases of MDR–TB decreased, but at a cost: New York City alone spent $175m over 4 years. The principal means of control has been "directly-observed therapy" (DOT), whereby patients are followed up for the whole of a long course of treatment, and are supervised every time they take their medicine. DOT has been a success in the

USA; but Dr Brennan at FDA told us that China has practised DOT since 1988 and still seems to have plenty of MDR–TB.

20. Dr Ginsberg does not consider the casebook closed. Whereas in 1991 MDR–TB was reported in only 13 States, it is now found in 42; and "There are still physicians out there who don't know the appropriate therapy". If political will falters and funding for public health measures falls away again, NIAID expect the problem to return. Dr Miller of CDC drew the moral: maintaining a proper public health infrastructure is much cheaper than managing the consequences of running it down.

21. UK and US scientists are working together to combat TB. Scientists at the Sanger Centre (funded by the Wellcome Trust) and the Institute for Genomic Research (funded by NIAID) are sequencing the TB genome; and the USA, the UK and France are contributing to a WHO working group on a vaccine against TB, which people at NIH regard as crucial to long-term success against this disease. (The BCG vaccine familiar in the UK is not recommended for use in the USA: it is regarded as ineffective and unnecessary, and it compromises a diagnostic technique widely used in the USA.)

22. In contrast, the pharmaceutical industry shows little interest in TB: the market is generally felt to be insufficient to justify developing new drugs; and firms with established drugs (e.g. quinolones) which might be effective against TB are reluctant to try them. We received three slightly different explanations for this reluctance. People at NIH put it down to fear that the long courses required for TB would throw up new side-effects; Dr Goldberger at FDA put it down to fear that a drug which became known as a TB drug would fall out of favour for other, more lucrative indications; Dr Siegfried at PhRMA reckoned that any drug which purported to be effective against resistant strains would be labelled so restrictively, at FDA's behest, that the market would be too small.

23. However Dr Goldberger knew of some pharmaceutical work in progress. CDC are experimenting with rifamycins; it is possible that this family of drugs may be effective over relatively short courses, which would improve compliance. And some manufacturers are working on drugs specifically for MDR–TB, on immunologic drugs to complement chemotherapy, and on vaccines. Dr Sheldon Morris of FDA told us that Merck Sharp and Dohme are making progress towards a DNA vaccine.

HIV/AIDS

24. Two special features of HIV are the virus's exceptional rate of mutation, so that resistance to any single drug evolves very quickly; and the exceptional success of activists in attracting resources to research. Of NIAID's 124 research projects in 1996, 50 concerned HIV.

25. The treatment currently favoured for HIV is "triple therapy", with three antivirals. According to people at PhRMA, even triple therapy gives rise to resistance after a time; and, with only ten drugs to choose from, only three non-overlapping regimens can be tried. However according to Dr Hu at CDC, a mutation which confers resistance to one drug sometimes opens up a target to another. People at NIH consider that the world's best hope for HIV, as for TB, is a vaccine; however according to Dr Livengood of the National Immunization Program this is a long way off.

Community Infections

Penicillin-resistant Streptococcus pneumoniae (PRP)

26. A major concern in the USA, more than in this country, is the rise in *Strep. pneumoniae* resistant to penicillins, cephalosporins and other drugs. Unlike hospital infections and TB, *Strep. pneumoniae* can affect anybody, including the healthy and wealthy; it may only cause a transient middle-ear infection or a cough, but it may also cause pneumonia, bacteraemia or meningitis. Drug-resistant *Strep. pneumoniae*, as a proportion of all isolates in a survey of US hospitals, rose rapidly from 3.6 per cent in 1987 to 14.5 per cent in 1994 (source: NIAID Profile 1996). In 1995, 23.6 per cent of all *Strep. pneumoniae* was resistant to penicillin, and a further 14.1 per cent had reduced susceptibility; more recent figures go up to 46 per cent, and even higher in children (source: Dr Heyse, NIAID). The rise in resistance has been matched in the USA by a rise in virulence (i.e. more invasive infections).

27. A substantial proportion of PRP has multi-drug resistance. According to Dr Schwartz of CDC, 7 per cent of *Strep. pneumoniae* is resistant to all oral antibiotics, and some strains are susceptible only to vancomycin. Vancomycin-resistant *Strep. pneumoniae* would be a very serious public health problem.

28. The rise in PRP in the USA is universally ascribed to over-prescription of antibiotics, particularly for upper respiratory tract infections ("Strep throat"), and for children with otitis media (middle-ear infection), but also for conditions such as acute bronchitis or a common cold where antibiotics are of no use at all. In the UK GPs usually give an ear infection 1–2 days to clear up before prescribing, but in the USA antibiotics are usually given at once. This is partly for fear of litigation, and partly due to pressure from patients and parents: see below. According to Dr Levy, for every case of otitis media where an antibiotic is justified, there are 10 where it is not.

29. The rise of PRP has prompted a search for a better *Strep. pneumoniae* vaccine, and a conjugate vaccine is now under trial. Dr Gorbach in Boston observed that an effective Strep vaccine, with the existing Hib vaccine, would all but eliminate bacterial otitis media, and thereby remove the biggest single cause of inappropriate prescribing in the USA.

30. PRP has recently been made notifiable in several States.

OTHER INFECTIONS

31. Dr Levy agreed that the infections noted above are the biggest threats to public health in the short term. For the longer term, he drew attention to *Neisseria gonorrhoeae*: in the USA, resistance to penicillin and tetracycline reached 31.6 per cent in 1995, and strains resistant to fluoroquinolones were found. He also mentioned Klebsiella and Pseudomonas.

Food-borne infections

32. As in the UK, the principal food-borne infections in the USA are Salmonella, *Campylobacter jejuni* and *Escherichia coli* (*E. coli*). Penta-resistant *Salmonella typhimurium* DT104 is on the increase; in 1996 it accounted for 33 per cent of Salmonella found in people, and 10.5 per cent in animals.

33. As noted above, the USA is as concerned about food poisoning as is the UK. The emphasis is different: whereas UK concern is focussed on home-produced meat, in the USA there is equal concern about imported fruit and vegetables. In 1996, the Department of Agriculture introduced Hazard Analysis at Critical Control Points (HACCP) regulations for slaughter-houses and chicken-houses: as someone at NIH put it, this means "microbiology instead of sniffing carcasses". There are proposals to create a unified "plough-to-plate" food safety agency, bringing together responsibilities currently divided between the Department of Agriculture and the FDA; the National Academy of Sciences is to report on this matter in August 1998.

34. People at NIH stressed the importance of extending epidemiology onto the farm. According to William James, the FSIS has made a start: in 1995 they tested 1,000 animals, and in 1996 2,000. Most of these were casualty animals, and therefore would not normally enter the food chain. However from this year on they intend to sample each year 20,000 animals which would normally enter the food chain.

35. Many of those whom we met agreed that antibiotics are overused in animal husbandry, and also in arboriculture and aquaculture (fish-farming). See below.

Parasites

36. Dr Colley and his colleagues at CDC told us about their work on parasitic infections.

(i) *Malaria* They speculated that the currently fashionable strategy of impregnating bednets may eventually induce resistance.

(ii) *Human helminths* There is no resistance problem yet; but new programmes of targeted mass treatment of children may create one.

(iii) *Headlice* There is anecdotal evidence of resistance, and no public-domain research. Treatment manufacturers blame parents for inadequate treatment.

(iv) *Vaginitis* The USA is experiencing some resistance of *Trichomonas vaginalis* to metronidazole, which is widely used in UK hospitals as a prophylactic in general abdominal surgery.

FIGHTING RESISTANCE

Surveillance

37. There is no shortage of information in the USA about infectious diseases and antimicrobial usage. Hospitals, health management organisations (HMOs) and pharmaceutical companies have plenty of data. However, as in the UK, standards and IT systems are not all compatible; and, unlike the UK, there is no network of national laboratories. Public health laboratories are the responsibility of the State or locality; the States are also responsible for deciding what conditions are notifiable, and their lists are not the same. Federal agencies therefore proceed by encouraging voluntary data-sharing, and convergence of standards around the National Committee for Clinical Laboratory Standards (NCCLS) and of software around WHONET.

38. A recent Institute of Medicine workshop on surveillance identified two desiderata: data must include locality, since resistance is often due to local phenomena; and it must include clinical outcome. Those we met at the Institute acknowledged that the ideal surveillance system has not been realised anywhere.

39. At CDC we learned from Mr Jarvis and his colleagues about the National Nosocomial Infection Surveillance (NNIS) system, and about Project ICARE (Intensive Care Antibiotic Resistance Epidemiology). NNIS began in 1970, as a voluntary system to collect demographic and infection data from certain wards in participating hospitals. It now involves 250 hospitals, all of 100 beds or more; it is still expanding, and becoming more representative of the generality of US hospitals. NNIS is confidential; CDC returns to each hospital its own results, in relation to the overall distribution.

40. ICARE takes NNIS data and adds information about antibiotic usage. It currently involves 40 hospitals, each of which receives a nominal $3–4000 to support data collection; it covers 13 "bug-drug" combinations, chosen for their clinical importance. Like NNIS, ICARE is confidential; CDC returns to each hospital its own results, in relation to the overall distribution. In feeding back results to each hospital, the ICARE team at CDC try to identify interventions which can bring down rates of resistance. "One size doesn't fit all": two hospitals may have equally high levels of MRSA; in one case the cause may turn out to be overuse of cephalosporins, in the other proximity to a nursing home with poor infection control. Dr John McGowan commented that, as a means of tackling resistance, ICARE has the advantage, over general guidelines, of being highly specific and taking full account of local circumstances, including constraints on resources.

41. One limiting factor for ICARE, admitted by CDC, is the usage data; if pharmacy information exists at all, it is often set up to inform billing rather than to analyse usage. Another, pointed out by Dr McGowan, is the absence of community surveillance, which for some bug-drug combinations would be crucial.

42. We were most impressed by ICARE, and wondered how the concept might be transplanted to the UK. Without external funds, probably only two or three UK hospitals would be interested. One way forward might be for a few UK hospitals to ask to participate in ICARE itself; alternatively, a free-standing UK project might be supported from the NHS R&D Budget.

Diagnostic testing

43. Many of our witnesses in the UK have called for the development of rapid tests for susceptibility and resistance. Dr Shively of FDA told us that there are several rapid susceptibility tests on the market (e.g. Vitek, MicroScan). The Crystal MRSA is an example of a rapid test for identifying MRSA, which uses a fluorescent signal; because it is a single test unit, the cost per test would be higher than using a susceptibility panel.

44. NIAID's recent "programme announcement" (i.e. call for proposals) on antibiotic resistance includes a challenge to develop rapid tests for susceptibility and resistance. Dr Ginsberg believed that rapid tests based on gene sequencing might still be 5 years away (Dr Gorbach said 10); however in the short term techniques were emerging based on the rate of bacterial growth. Dr Shively showed us the ESP Culture System, used for detecting positive blood cultures and

mycobacterial growth in broth cultures; it is based on detecting pressure changes due to gas consumption or gas production when bacteria metabolize. Such systems have potential for being used for TB susceptibility testing. Bacteriophages also present possibilities for diagnosis—though not necessarily for treatment, according to those we met at NIAID.

45. Dr O'Brien said that, with over 200 resistance genes already, to expect genetic tests for all of them might be unrealistic. Dr Shively suggested that, in any case, having rapid susceptibility test results may not affect how physicians use results. Although "rapid" tests give a faster turnaround time, the results are not available until bacteria in cultures are isolated. Thus "rapid" results are usually not available at the time antimicrobials are prescribed, as many patients are treated empirically. Physicians may not change already prescribed antimicrobials unless the patient fails to get better or has a life-threatening condition.

Hygiene and infection control

46. We heard little about infection control, perhaps because we visited no hospitals. Dr Heyse of NIAID identified a general "breakdown" in hygiene, infection control and public health programmes. There is a major campaign of public education in hand-washing—though Miss Stoiber of the US Department of Health suggested that this could amount to a form of "victim-blaming", and that other factors such as intensive food production were more important.

Pharmaceutical industry and new drug development

47. The people we met tended to be realistic about what could be expected from the pharmaceutical industry. Industry has "a different bottom line" from public health services; in the end, its priorities are bound to be market-driven.

48. It was observed at NIH that most new anti-infectives of recent years were really variations on a theme, rather than wholly novel drugs: e.g. there are 8 variants of vancomycin. Dr Rakowsky at FDA told us that the last new class of drugs, with a new target, came out in 1971. However industry has regained interest in anti-infectives, in the light of rising resistance and new scientific opportunities; and new classes are now under development.

49. Dr Levy of Tufts is actively researching mechanisms of resistance and new approaches to overcoming it. He mentioned three lines of investigation. First, in a joint venture, he is hoping to apply the tetracyclines (which fell out of general use in the 1970s) to combat MRSA/VRSA. Secondly, his team are looking for new gene targets. Finally, they are exploring "antipathogenesis". This involves agents which do not destroy the bacterium, but render it harmless, e.g. by neutralising toxins; since they apply no selective pressure, they ought not to give rise to resistance. Certain companies are interested.

50. Dr Levy also mentioned "probiotics", whereby beneficial or harmless bacteria are encouraged to displace pathogens and resistant strains. This approach is being used against malaria and its vectors, and Dr Levy believes that it may offer a substitute for animal growth promoters. Bacteriophages hold no promise for human medicine, he believes, but might have applications in arboriculture.

Commercial surveillance

51. In the USA, there are commercial companies which conduct disease surveillance and sell their results to pharmaceutical companies, to inform drug development and marketing strategies. As Dr Siegfried of PhRMA pointed out, information which shows that an established drug is slowly losing its effect is bound to be commercially sensitive.

Genomics

52. In the long term, the future of both diagnosis and treatment may depend on understanding the genes responsible for infection and resistance. At PhRMA, we were told that industry is researching this area intensively. Several commercial companies have already sequenced the genome of MRSA, but the information is not in the public domain; so NIH are funding a separate non-commercial sequencing project. They are funding a further 11 genome sequencing projects, including TB and the enterococcus, with a total estimated budget of $5m for 1997.

53. Of NIAID's 124 research projects with a primary emphasis on antimicrobial resistance in 1996, 47 concerned genetic aspects of resistance; but people at NIH said that, though having the data was exciting, it was not yet clear how best to use it. Dr Levin suggested that genomic treatments would be so specific as to be of doubtful commercial viability.

USE OF ANTIMICROBIALS

Prescribing practice

54. The prescribing practices of individual physicians (GPs) are no less significant a driver of resistance in the USA than in the UK; but in the USA the government has even less control. Who pays the piper calls the tune; in the USA, the government pays for healthcare only for the old (Medicare) and the poor (Medicaid). The rest is paid for by insurers or by the patients themselves; and the government has no locus to regulate practice. FDA has some control over drug use by regulation of labelling: physicians who authorise "off-label" use open themselves to suits for negligence. However, as Dr Rakowsky told us, if labelling were too restrictive, industry would be discouraged from developing drugs at all.

55. CDC put the level of unnecessary use of antibiotics in the community at 20–50 per cent, and in hospital at 25–45 per cent.

56. Managed care (see below) is affecting practice, but whether for good or ill was not clear. As Miss Stoiber of the US Department of Health saw it, on the one hand, managed care was squeezing cross-subsidies for local and State public health services; on the other hand, HMOs have a shared interest with public health services in ensuring rational treatment and curbing over-prescribing. Dr Siegfried of PhRMA was less ambivalent: managed care strains the patient's confidence in the doctor, and pressures the doctor to give less time to the patient; both factors favour prescribing over not prescribing. To transpose these arguments from the USA to the UK, for "managed care" read "the NHS internal market".

57. Everyone we met agreed that achieving rational or "prudent" use of antibiotics depends very largely on education and persuasion of physicians and their patients. Dr Rakowsky pointed to some of the difficulties of educating physicians: antibiotics are beguilingly safe to prescribe in terms of direct risk to the patient—though not in terms of long-term risk to public or indeed individual health; antibiotic use is scantily covered in undergraduate lecture courses, and most subsequent education is from "the guy who gives you the pizza and the pen", the pharmaceutical salesman or "detailman". Dr Siegfried of PhRMA defended the industry: free gifts are out of fashion; the detailman should be seen as an educator; what physicians do with the information is ultimately up to them; and in many cases the detailman must now make his pitch not just to the physician, but to the HMO which imposes on all its physicians a restricted formulary.

58. Dr Goldberger of FDA drew attention to one common pattern of bad practice. A patient is given a broad-spectrum antibiotic pending diagnosis. Diagnosis then reveals that a narrow-spectrum drug would be appropriate; but the prescription is not changed.

59. Dr Mark Lipsic, a colleague of Dr Levin from Emory University examined some of the "rules of thumb" which tend to guide doctors prescribing antibiotics:

- (i) *Finish the course* This may or may not be good advice, depending on the effect on the commensal flora.
- (ii) *Give several drugs in combination* The effectiveness of multi-drug therapies is well attested for TB and HIV.
- (iii) *If the regimen is failing, do not simply add one more drug* This is proven.
- (iv) *Give different drugs in rotation* The evidence in favour of "drug cycling" is anecdotal; it may in fact be counter-productive.

He showed how practical questions of this sort can be addressed by population biology and mathematical modelling.

60. Dr John McGowan of Emory University told us how, in May this year, Canada held a national meeting of all those with a stake in the issue, and agreed a national plan to reduce medical use of antibiotics by 23 per cent over 3 years, by concentrating mainly on mis-prescription for upper

respiratory tract infections. The government has agreed to fund the plan. "The USA should have done this years ago," said Dr McGowan; so, perhaps, should the UK.

61. We listened out for stories of resistance rates actually being brought down, and found only three. One is the story of MDR–TB, told above. The second comes from Finland, where use of erythromycin for streptococcal infections rose sharply in the late 1980s, causing a rise in resistance from 5 per cent in 1988 to 19 per cent in 1993. A national warning was issued, with recommendations on alternative drugs. Use of erythromycin fell by half; and by 1996 the rate of resistance was down to 8.6 per cent. The third was told by Dr Gorbach in Boston: one hospital eliminated second and third generation cephalosporins from its formulary, and halved its rate of VRE. Dr Gorbach knew of no other such stories. Dr Bennish of Boston pointed out that the premise of such stories, and of our efforts to control resistance, is that selective pressure is the main driver of resistance. This may not be true in all cases, and removing the selective pressure may only rarely result in the return of susceptible strains.

Pressure from patients

62. In the USA perhaps even more than in the UK, many patients expect their doctor to prescribe, and will be reluctant to leave the surgery until he has done so. Education must therefore not be confined to the doctor, but must also reach the patient. Several of those we met cited seatbelts, red meat and smoking to show that public attitudes can be changed by campaigns of public health education.

Pressure from parents

63. It came out time and again that much of the pressure on US physicians to prescribe antibiotics comes from the parents of poorly children. Even more mothers go out to work in the USA than in the UK, and cannot easily take time off to look after a sick child; and some daycare centres (nurseries) even require a certificate that antibiotics have been taken before a child who has been sick is allowed to return. According to Miss Shoemaker of the American Society for Microbiology, the number of US children under 6 attending daycare has risen to 60 per cent since 1975; over that period, the amount of antibiotics prescribed has tripled, and 20–25 per cent of antibiotics now prescribed in the USA are prescribed for children. Daycare centres are also, of course, an ideal setting for the spread of infection.

64. All this may carry warnings for the UK, where public policy has for years favoured the out-to-work parent and encouraged childcare outside the home.

Education for prudent use

65. Dr Levin of Emory University observed that prudent use requires that the patient's immediate perceived need be subordinated to the wider interests of public health. This will only happen if the costs and consequences of imprudent use are better documented than at present, and if it can be shown by evaluation that imprudent use may even harm the patient. He pointed out that cultural factors are sometimes on the side of the angels: for instance, in Italy antibiotics are believed to stunt children's growth.

66. Dr Levy of Tufts agreed as to the importance of sound cost-benefit analysis. Dr Schwartz of CDC and Dr Bennish of Boston both believe they can show that previous treatment with antibiotics is a risk factor for infection with resistant strains.

67. Dr Schwartz has worked on educating community physicians and their patients, with a view to controlling the rise of PRP (see above). In focus groups, physicians acknowledged overusing antibiotics by as much as 50 per cent. They blamed pressure from patients, and shortage of consultation time: it is quicker to prescribe, than to explain why a prescription would be inappropriate. Dr Schwartz has therefore produced the following aids for physicians: professional information sheets; a simple patient information leaflet for the waiting room, explaining that unnecessary antibiotics are bad for the patient; a "non-prescription" form; Q&A sheets for parents; and a letter for parents to give to their child-carer. Pilot projects are now under way in five States; CDC is equipping the local health department to train senior doctors to disseminate the concepts and materials to their peers. Evaluation will show whether these approaches reduce inappropriate use, and whether this in turn affects the level of PRP. We asked whether the pharmaceutical industry had been supportive; Dr Schwartz has had practical help from SKB, and other firms have made encouraging noises.

68. Dr Avorn of Harvard Medical School has also worked on education for prudent use. His approach is modelled on that of the pharmaceutical industry, and not unlike that of Dr Schwartz. He began with focus groups of physicians. These revealed two groups of doctors: some who overprescribe out of ignorance; and others who consciously overprescribe in order to satisfy their patients. For the second group, like Dr Schwartz, he provides "paper placebos". For the first, he sends out "academic detailmen": pharmacists from the medical school who meet physicians one-to-one, on the same basis as salesmen, to talk about prudent prescribing. He has shown that every $1 spent on these actions saves $2 on the drugs bill. His approach has been taken up in various places around the USA; similar approaches have been tried in various parts of the UK, and adopted nationwide in Australia. He acknowledged that some doctors require to be persuaded that prudent use is not just a euphemism for cutting costs at the expense of patient care.

69. As a location for education of patients, Dr Avorn commended schools; so did Dr Levy. The Alliance for the Prudent Use of Antibiotics, which was set up in 1981 and now has members in 92 countries including a few in the UK, has produced material for schools. APUA also produces patient leaflets, issues a newsletter and organises conferences. It encountered initial hostility from the pharmaceutical industry, but this is wearing off.

70. The people we met over lunch in Boston disagreed as to the appropriate level of coercion. Dr Gorbach favours control, e.g. by requiring that every prescription for a drug associated with a resistance problem be accompanied by a "chit" giving the reason for prescribing. Dr Medeiros considers that this would restrict professional freedom to a degree unacceptable in the USA; he believes that, if surveillance is thorough and its findings are properly communicated, doctors will moderate their practice voluntarily. Dr Bennish inclines towards Dr Gorbach's position; he considers that Dr Medeiros underestimates the power of pharmaceutical advertising, and he would like to see such advertising controlled.

Length of course

71. We put it to the FDA that their policy encouraged pharmaceutical companies to specify longer courses of antibiotics than were necessary, thereby adding to the general antibiotic load. Dr Goldberger replied that the FDA has no policy on length of courses; it relies on the manufacturer to decide what length to use for the trials leading up to licensing, and licenses the the drug on that basis. Under pressure from managed care (see below) to reduce costs, manufacturers are beginning to try shorter courses as a way to gain market advantage; the FDA requires to be convinced in each case that the short course is at least as effective as the longer one. Dr Siegfried of PhRMA commented that the manufacturer's view of the ideal length of treatment often changes once a drug reaches the market.

Antibiotics in old people's homes

72. Nursing homes are big business in the USA, as in the UK. People at the Institute of Medicine said that they were under-regulated. Dr Siegfried at PhRMA drew attention to an invisible form of "drug abuse": informal and inappropriate pill-sharing by old people. ICARE staff at CDC told us of a case where the main source of resistant infections in a hospital turned out to be a nearby nursing home.

Antibiotics for export

73. We asked the FDA about regulation of antibiotics manufactured for export. Antibiotics manufactured in the USA for export to a country with lower standards are not required to meet the high standards set by the FDA for drugs intended for use by Americans. However drugs may not be exported which have passed their "sell-by" date.

Antibiotics in farming

74. "Antibiotic resistance is our most important issue just now," said Dr Stephen Sundlof, Director of the FDA Center for Veterinary Medicine; and its importance in the context of farming is recognised by politicians and the press.

75. The flashpoint is the fluoroquinolones. In 1995 the FDA approved the prescription of sarafloxacin for the prevention of pneumonia in poultry, subject to resistance monitoring up and down the food chain. There was apparently some ambiguity in this decision: Dr Levy, who was involved, was left with the impression that approval would be provisional, but it turned out not to

be. Then, early this year, a 'phone call from Colindale alerted FDA to the emergence of ciprofloxacin resistance in *S. typhimurium DT104* in the UK. Since then, FDA has issued no more approvals for fluoroquinolones for animals; meanwhile, sure enough, 10 per cent resistance to fluoroquinolones has been found in Campylobacter, though none as yet in Salmonella. FDA are using DNA fingerprinting to see whether resistance in Campylobacter can be traced to poultry and sarafloxacin; they suspect so strongly, but have not yet proved it.

76. FDA believe that lives are not at risk; but Dr Sundlof frankly admitted that they are not sure, and they are very concerned. At the same time, they have no intention to deprive agriculture altogether of the benefits of antibiotics; they have to balance the interests of agriculture against those of public health, and, as Dr Sundlof explained, this is not easy. Interestingly, he did not consider that this was an issue which could safely be put to the people. The FDA has seconded someone to the UK CVL and PHLS to learn from our experience of fluoroquinolone use. In discussion at FDA, someone took us aback by asking simply, why the UK continues to approve fluoroquinolones for animal use, when the USA has stopped doing so on advice from British scientists.

77. Dr Tauxe expressed to us CDC's serious concern over continued veterinary use of fluoroquinolones. He told us how Congress recently blew a large hole in the Swann regime by legislating to permit any antibiotic approved for use in one species, including man, to be used in any other. This enactment was promoted by the veterinary profession; it was resisted by CDC, who succeeded only in winning exceptions for the fluoroquinolones and the glycopeptides.

78. US agriculture uses around 16m lb of antimicrobials for animals every year, of which CDC believes 40–80 per cent to be unnecessary. In Dr Tauxe's view, antibiotics are being used as a "crutch" for otherwise impossibly intensive farming practices. He likened the modern farm to a nineteenth-century city before the revolution in sanitation and public health. He pointed to the example of Denmark, where by improved farming practice the level of Salmonella had been dramatically reduced without increasing costs.

79. Like the EU, the FDA has prohibited the growth promoter avoparcin. Dr Sundlof was unable to reveal the reason, but said that it was not fear of fostering resistance to other glycopeptides including vancomycin, though this fear would now deter the FDA from approving animal use of any glycopeptide. The USA has plenty of vancomycin-resistant bacteria as it is (see above, VISA and VRE). Dr Sundlof blames this on overuse of vancomycin in human medicine; but Dr Siegfried of PhRMA, who is personally "appalled" at the amount of antibiotics fed to animals, believes that there is significant illegal use of vancomycin in US agriculture, while Dr Levy believes that VRE originally reached the USA from Europe.

80. We raised at FDA the case of virginiamycin, which was approved for animal use before human use of cognate antibiotics became a possibility. Dr Sundlof replied that the FDA could not block all veterinary drugs for fear of compromising possible human uses of substances cognate to the drug in question but as yet undeveloped. They are trying to find ways to predict resistance in advance of approval, by examining data from clinical trials; but these are of limited predictive value. As Dr Sundlof put it, such cases present a "difficult regulatory challenge"; Dr Levy regards this issue as a major weakness in the Swann regime.

81. Until 1991, FDA approved most animal drugs for sale over the counter. All approvals since then have been for prescription only. The most vocal protesters have been the fish-farmers. We encountered widespread concern about the use of antibiotics in aquaculture (fish-farming); Dr Levy commended Norway for best practice in moving from overuse of antibiotics towards vaccines.

82. Several of those we met commended the conclusion of the recent WHO meeting on this issue in Berlin, that growth promoters should be progressively removed from the agricultural scene. Dr Levy described the meeting as a "historic moment". In his view, the low-level long-term use of growth promoters is much more damaging than veterinary prophylaxis. He told us how Sweden banned all growth promoters at a stroke, without destroying Swedish agriculture. Sweden is a rich country, with a highly centralised agricultural industry; Dr Levy acknowledged that such a step would be much harder for, say, China. The agricultural industry has for too long "refused to admit that we are on the same planet", and hidden behind the difficulty of proving that resistant strains induced in animals are the same as those which cause human disease (the "show me a dead body"

argument)—though Dr Levy has proved this to his own satisfaction in the case of *E. coli*. The Berlin meeting was particularly important because it included industry representatives.

Resistance markers in genetically modified organisms (GMOs)

83. Dr Beru of FDA gave us the US position on resistance markers in GMOs. The FDA adopted a regulatory policy in 1992. For foods derived from GMOs, FDA believes evaluation of resistance markers should be based on three questions:

(i) How toxic is the enzyme generated by virtue of the resistance gene?
(ii) Could the enzyme act directly on antibiotics?
(iii) Could resistance be transferred from the GMO?

84. The first case to come forward was the "Flavr Savr" tomato. The enzyme was not toxic, and could not act directly. There was a very remote possibility of transfer; but even in the worst case scenario the effect would have been trivial. After 4 years of review, the tomato was approved. Since then FDA has finalised consultations on 30 GMOs, mostly with resistance markers, all of them plants. One was Ciba-Geigy's GM maize, which was also approved by the EU; the UK ACNFP approved it for processed products but not for unprocessed products.

Biocides in domestic articles

85. Dr Levy drew our attention to the new phenomenon of domestic articles—kitchenware, soap, even children's toys—which are advertised as containing antibacterials. To the extent that this is true, he regards it as a further serious threat to normal bacterial ecology. Such products appeared in the USA in 1995, and are just beginning to appear in the UK.[2]

TO SEE OURSELVES AS OTHERS SEE US

86. People we met were generally coy about commenting on the UK's performance in the fight against resistance; some frankly admitted to knowing little about the UK scene. Dr Levy suggested that the UK was perhaps a little complacent, possibly because rates of the main resistant strains are lower than in the USA. Regarding antibiotics for animals, he suggested that the UK had relied on the Swann regime for too long; as noted above, we were challenged at FDA on the licensing of enrofloxacin.

87. Over lunch in Boston, Dr O'Brien spoke highly of PHLS's system for surveillance of Salmonella, which drew early attention to the problem of *S. typhimurium DT104*; and Dr Medeiros and Dr Gorbach observed that the UK has tools of control which the USA lacks, e.g. the NHS, the British National Formulary, the prescribing data compiled by the Prescription Pricing Authority, and a culture less averse to regulation.

"TAKE-HOME MESSAGES"

88. The following are the messages which came over to us most strongly during the visit:

(i) Antimicrobial resistance can be seen as a subset of a series of threats to public health posed by emerging and re-emerging infections. (See above, paragraph 5.)

(ii) UK hospitals should expect before long to have as much trouble with VRE as US hospitals do already. (Paragraph 15.)

(iii) The USA has paid a heavy price, in money and lives, for letting down her guard against TB; the UK must not make the same mistake. (Paragraph 17.)

(iv) Multi-resistant *Strep pneumoniae* poses a most serious threat to public health outside the hospital, and the search for better vaccines is urgent. (Paragraph 26.)

(v) A surveillance system along the lines of ICARE would be a great asset to UK hospitals. (Paragraph 40.)

---

2 See the evidence of the Royal Pharmaceutical Society (p 457) and the British Association for Chemical Specialities (p 545).

(vi) The key to controlling resistance is prudent use of antibiotics; and the key to prudent use is education—of policy-makers, professionals and the public. (Paragraph 57.)

(vii) As pre-school childcare becomes ever more prevalent in the UK, we should be mindful of the implications for the spread of infection and the use of antibiotics. (Paragraph 63.)

(viii) It is possible, and cost-effective, to educate and equip doctors to change their prescribing practices. (Paragraphs 67, 68.)

(ix) The licensing of enrofloxacin for animal use may have been a grave mistake, which must not be repeated. (Paragraphs 75, 76.)

SOULSBY OF SWAFFHAM PRIOR
5 December 1997

DIARY

MONDAY 17TH NOVEMBER, WASHINGTON

National Institutes of Health (NIH)
National Institute of Allergy and Infectious Diseases (NIAID)

1. NIH is the US equivalent of the MRC. Within NIH, NIAID is responsible for conducting and supporting research into infectious diseases. NIAID's research budget for 1996 was $31m. We met:

- Dr Dennis Dixon, Chief of the Bacteriology and Mycology Branch
- Dr Amar Bhat, Programme Officer for Europe
- Dr Ann Ginsberg, Medical and Program Officer for TB, Leprosy and other Mycobacterial Diseases
- Dr Stephen Heyse, Medical Bacteriology and Antibacterial Resistance Program Officer
- Dr David Klein, Respiratory Diseases Officer
- Dr Dennis Long, Bacterial and Viral Enteric Diseases Program Officer
- Linda Scott, Policy Analysis Branch

2. At the end of a wide-ranging discussion, we asked what were the top priorities in the fight against resistance. The answers were: genomics; vaccine development, especially for TB and HIV; epidemiology on the farm; and "Wash your hands!"

Ambassador's lunch

3. Over lunch at the Ambassador's Residence, we met, among others:

- Dr Gail Cassell, Vice President of Infectious Diseases Research, Eli Lilly
- Donna Vogt, of the Congressional Research Service Science Policy Division
- Janet Shoemaker, Director of Public and Scientific Affairs, American Society for Microbiology
- Miss Stoiber, of the US Department of Health and Human Services
- Dr Polly Harrison, Institute of Medicine

4. In discussion around the table, Dr Cassell stressed the importance of infectious diseases to the USA and to the world; and particularly the issue of food poisoning. She called for public and professional education, and for control of antibiotic use in farming. Miss Vogt indicated that Congress is well seized of the significance of food poisoning. Miss Shoemaker stressed the over-prescription of antibiotics to children, and the importance of basic hygiene. Dr Harrison noted that very worrying links are emerging between infections and chronic disease, for example cardiovascular disease and some cancers.

5. Miss Stoiber drew attention to the growth of "**managed care**", whereby commercial "health management organisations" (HMOs) manage the healthcare of people with health insurance with a view to controlling cost to the insurers. The government is not involved in managed care, though during our visit the President announced a plan for a "Patient's Bill of Rights", a voluntary code for HMOs which may be modelled on the UK Patient's Charter. Miss Stoiber also mentioned food poisoning, for which she blamed intensive farming practices more than poor hygiene in the home.

White House Office of Science and Technology Policy (OSTP)

6. OSTP is the US equivalent of OST; it is led by the President's Science Advisor, Dr Jack Gibbons, as OST is headed by the Chief Scientific Adviser, Sir Robert May. Its functions are advisory and managerial rather than executive. We met:

- Dr Laura Efros, Senior Research Analyst
- Rachel Levinson, Assistant Director for Life Sciences

Conversation turned mainly on the recent Presidential Directive on emerging infections.

National Academy of Sciences Institute of Medicine

7. The National Academy of Sciences is the US equivalent of the Royal Society; the Institute of Medicine is its medical wing. We met:

- Dr Polly Harrison, Director, Forum on Emerging Infections, Institute of Medicine
- Philip Russell, Professor of International Health, Johns Hopkins University
- Stephen Morse, Assistant Professor of Epidemiology, Columbia University
- William James, Food Safety Inspection Service, US Department of Agriculture
- Andrew Pope, Senior Staff Officer, Institute of Medicine
- Rick Manning, Senior Program Officer, Institute of Medicine
- Tania Williams, Program Officer, National Academy of Sciences

8. They told us about the Institute's report "Emerging Infections" of 1992, and actions to follow it up. The CDC produced a national plan, which has attracted Congressional funding, and established ICARE (see above). The American Society for Microbiology set up a task force on surveillance. The Institute itself established the Forum on Emerging Infections; the Forum has held two workshops, on encouraging drug development ("Orphans and Incentives") and on "Antimicrobial Resistance, Surveillance and Response". Another is planned, on the implications of changes in US healthcare; and an interdisciplinary project on the ecology and evolution of infections is being launched.

TUESDAY 18TH NOVEMBER, WASHINGTON

Food and Drug Administration (FDA)

9. The FDA regulates food and drugs. Their role is essentially passive: when a company applies for something to be licensed for certain uses, FDA decides whether to license it or not; but it is not their role to suggest improvements to the product, or alternative indications for use. However they have a research programme for vaccines. We met:

- Donald Aronson, Associate Director for Europe;
- Dr Mark Goldberger, Director, Division of Special Pathogens and Immunologic Drug Products, Center for Drug Evaluation and Research (CDER), who talked about TB;
- Dr Alex Rakowsky, Division of Anti-Infective Drug Products, CDER, who described the FDA's systems for **accelerated and emergency drug approval**, and for **Orphan Drug** designation. Accelerated approval does not in itself reduce time to market by more than one or two years; much more time can be saved if the manufacturer is prepared to take the business risks of running trials simultaneously rather than in sequence, and of committing manufacturing capacity in anticipation, and if the patient community are prompt to enrol for clinical trials. The Orphan Drug system was set up in

1992 to encourage development of drugs with a potential US market of fewer than 200,000 patients p.a.; threats in Congress to rewrite the rules had a "chilling" effect, and put industry off the scheme;

- Dr Michael Brennan, Chief, Laboratory of Mycobacteriology, Center for Biologics Evaluation and Research, and his colleague Dr Sheldon Morris, who covered TB vaccines;

- Dr Stephen Sundlof, Director, Center for Veterinary Medicine, who spoke mainly about animal use of the fluoroquinolones. He set out the difference between the FDA's approaches to regulating human and animal drugs. **The FDA puts people ahead of animals**. Therefore, whereas with human drugs benefits may outweigh costs, drugs for food animals must show "reasonable certainty of no harm" to humans, regardless of benefits to the animal;

- Dr Linda Tollefson, Director of Surveillance and Compliance, Center for Veterinary Medicine;

- Dr Nega Beru, Consumer Safety Officer, Center for Food Safety and Applied Nutrition, who spoke about resistance markers in GMOs;

- Roxanne Shively, Division of Clinical Laboratory Devices, Center for Devices and Radiological Health.

Pharmaceutical Research and Manufacturers of America (PhRMA)

10. PhRMA is the US analogue of the ABPI, except that it embraces only manufacturers who conduct R&D in the USA, and excludes purely generic producers. We met DrJohn Siegfried, Deputy Vice President for Regulatory and Scientific Affairs, and Dr Gillian Woollett, Assistant Vice President Biologics and Biotechnology.

WEDNESDAY 19TH NOVEMBER, ATLANTA

Centers for Disease Prevention and Control (CDC)

11. We were welcomed first by Dr Claire Broom, Deputy Director of CDC. She explained that CDC supports the States in their responsibilities for public health. It conducts and supports applied research (basic research is the responsibility of NIH); it designs, manages and evaluates surveillance programmes, and receives notice of notifiable conditions; it gives grants to the States for public health programmes, and steers such programmes by means including guidance, targets (e.g. for disease reduction or vaccine coverage), incentive funds and league tables. CDC staff are to be found in the health department of every state. CDC's UK counterpart is PHLS.

12. We were also welcomed by Dr Jim Hughes, Director of the National Center for Infectious Diseases, and colleagues.

13. Next we met Dr Bruce Levin and colleagues, from Emory University School of Medicine. Dr Levin's field is population biology; he finds antibiotic resistance interesting in its own right, since it shows evolution in action. He gave us his reasons for believing that **resistance is a one-way street**: even if antibiotic use were cut back sharply, resistance would wane slowly if at all; even moderate use still imposes heavy selective pressure; and, if use were resumed then resistance would rise again more rapidly than before. As he put it, "We are committed to an arms race"; disarmament is not an option. He contemplated a future without effective antibiotics: infectious diseases could still be controlled by traditional means, as they were before the 1940s; but transplants, cancer chemotherapy and other modern medical techniques which depend on antibiotics would be impossible.

14. Then, from the Division of Bacterial and Mycotic Diseases, we met Dr Mitchell Cohen, Director, Dr Ben Schwartz, and Dr Robert Tauxe, Medical Officer.

15. We were entertained to lunch at the Houston Mill House by the National Foundation for the CDC: Charlie Stokes, Executive Director; Subie Green, Director of Development; and Nicole Kruse, Development Officer. The Foundation raises funds to help CDC to operate on the edges of its mandate, by supporting pilot projects, overseas projects, health education, IT, international

fellowships etc. It has no analogue in the UK; some of what it does would fall to the major medical charities.

16. From the Division of Parasitic Diseases, we then met Dr Daniel Colley, Director, Dr Peter Schantz (once a pupil of Lord Soulsby at the University of Maryland), Dr William Collins, Dr Trenton Ruebush and Dr Peter Bloland.

17. Finally we met Robert Baldwin, Assistant Director for International Health Liaison. He explained that CDC has no mandate to work overseas; when they do so, it is therefore on a consultancy basis, by invitation.

THURSDAY 20TH NOVEMBER, ATLANTA

Centers for Disease Prevention and Control (CDC) (continued)

18. From the Hospital Infections Program, we met William Jarvis, Director, and Dr Lennox Archibald.

19. From the National Center for HIV, STD and TB Prevention, we met Dr Bess Miller, Dr Todd Weber, Dr Dale Hu and Dr Marisa Moore.

20. We then met Dr John Livengood, Director, and colleagues from the National Immunization Program. They discussed the paradox that, if a vaccine is successful, the rate of disease may fall below the rate of adverse reaction to the vaccine, provoking an irrational loss of public confidence.

21. Over lunch we also met Dr John McGowan, Professor of Infectious Diseases at Emory University.

22. Our visit to CDC was meticulously organised by Linda Ford, Chief of International Visitors Activity. We were surprised to find that CDC is in part a uniformed service.

BOSTON

Consul-General's dinner

23. Over dinner at the Somerset Club, kindly hosted by Mr Jim Poston, HM Consul-General, we met Dr Stuart Levy, Director of the Center for Adaptation Genetics and Drug Resistance at Tufts University School of Medicine and founding President of the international Alliance for the Prudent Use of Antibiotics; and Dr Thomas O'Brien, Medical Director of the Microbiology Laboratory at Brigham and Women's Hospital, Director of the WHO Collaborating Center in Boston, and creator of WHONET.

24. Dr Levy, a lively and long-standing campaigner on this issue, expressed delight that it was receiving attention at Westminster. He declared himself an optimist—if only because, in the USA, the present position is so bad that major improvement would be relatively easy to achieve.

25. Dr O'Brien expressed "amazement" at the ability of bacteria to evolve. He regards the recent emergence of 2–300 resistance genes, under the artificial selective pressure of antibiotics, as an evolutionary "disorder". The challenge, as he sees it, is to mobilize the information about resistance which microbiologists already have.

FRIDAY 21ST NOVEMBER, BOSTON

Alliance for the Prudent Use of Antibiotics (APUA)

26. In the Sackler Library at Tufts University we met Dr Levy again, and colleagues from APUA.

Working lunch

27. Over lunch, we met Dr Levy; Dr O'Brien; Dr Michael Bennish, Associate Professor of Paediatrics at Tufts University; Dr Anton Medeiros, Professor at Brown University School of Medicine; and Dr Sherwood Gorbach, Professor of Immunology, Molecular Biology, Microbiology and Community Health at Tufts University.

28. Finally, after lunch, we met Dr Jerry Avorn, Assistant Professor of Medicine at Harvard Medical School, who told us about his work on doctor and patient behaviour.

APPENDIX 7

Some important antimicrobial agents

Agent	Principal applications
β–lactams	
Penicillin	Streptococci, pneumococci
Flucloxacillin/cloxacillin/methicillin	Staphylococci
Ampicillin/amoxycillin ± clavulanate	Staphylococci, streptococci, pneumococci, plus common respiratory and enteric organisms
Cephalosporins (1st, 2nd and 3rd generations)	As above, with enhanced stability to β–lactamases and hospital pathogens; broad spectrum
Carbapenems (e.g. imipenem)	Very broad spectrum activity against hospital pathogens
Macrolides Erythromycin, clarithromycin, azithromycin and others	Streptococci, pneumococci, Legionella etc (± staphylococci)
Fluoroquinolones (also known simply as quinolones) Ciprofloxacin and many more	Enteric, urinary and respiratory tract pathogens; used also for hospital infections
Aminoglycosides	
Streptomycin	TB
Gentamicin and amikacin	Broad spectrum: hospital pathogens including *Pseudomonas aeruginosa*
Glycopeptides Vancomycin and teicoplanin	MRSA, enterococci
Rifamycins Rifampicin and others	TB; prophylaxis against meningococcal disease
Miscellaneous anti-TB agents Isoniazid, pyrazinamide, ethambutol	TB
Folate inhibitors Trimethoprim ± sulphonamides ('Septrin')	Urinary tract infections (some in respiratory tract disease)
Streptogramins	Being developed against MRSA and enterococci
Oxazolidinones	Being developed against MRSA and enterococci

APPENDIX 8

Glossary

Bacteriophage: a virus that attacks bacteria. Each bacteriophage acts specifically against a particular species of bacterium.

Bacterium: microscopic single-celled organism, which may or may not be a pathogen.

Clostridium difficile: a bacterium which can cause severe diarrhoea or enterocolitis. This most commonly occurs following a course of antibiotics which has disturbed the normal bacterial flora of the patient's gut.

Colonisation: when micro-organisms reside on living tissue without causing disease.

Community: refers to diseases or health services which occur outside hospitals.

Compliance: the degree to which patients follow the instructions for taking a course of treatment.

Consultant in Communicable Disease Control (CCDC): a doctor, appointed by each Health Authority, who has responsibility for the surveillance, prevention and control of infections in the community.

DNA: deoxyribonucleic acid. The genetic material of nearly all living organisms, which controls heredity and is located in the cell nucleus,

Empirical treatment: management of disease, such as drug treatment, based on experience or observation rather than laboratory investigations, x-rays etc.

Enterococcus: a bacterium commonly associated with bladder, skin and wound infections.

Epidemiology: the study of the occurrence, cause, control and prevention of disease in populations, as opposed to individuals.

Escherichia coli (E.coli): bacterium commonly associated with a wide range of infections, including bladder infections and diarrhoea.

Flora: micro-organisms which normally reside on the skin, in the gut and in the mouth and upper respiratory tract. They usually protect these tissues from diseases.

Gonococcus: a bacterium which is the cause of gonorrhoea, a sexually transmitted disease.

Haemophilus influenzae: a bacterium which most commonly causes respiratory tract infections and meningitis.

Helminth: any of the parasitic worms including flukes, tapeworms and nematodes.

Immunocompetent: having normal immune responses, as in a normal healthy person.

Immunosuppressed: having impaired immunity due to disease, for example cancer, or treatment, for example steroid drugs or radiotherapy.

In vitro: tests undertaken in laboratory apparatus, for example test tubes, not in a living human or animal. Literally, "in the glass".

In vivo: tests undertaken within a living human or animal. Literally, "in the living being".

Meningococcus: a bacterium which most commonly causes meningitis and septicaemia or blood-poisoning.

Microbe: any organism too small to be visible to the naked eye. Micro-organisms include bacteria, fungi, viruses and protozoa.

Microbiology: the science of the isolation and identification of micro-organisms. Medical microbiology is concerned with those micro-organisms which cause disease in humans.

Morbidity: disease, as opposed to mortality (death).

Mycobacterium tuberculosis: a bacterium which is the cause of tuberculosis (TB).

Pathogen: a micro-organism that can cause disease.

Pertussis: whooping cough. An acute infection, usually of childhood, which has characteristic spasms of coughing.

Pneumococcus: a bacterium most commonly associated with pneumonia and meningitis.

Prophylaxis: any means taken to prevent disease. For example, vaccination, or giving antibiotics when patients undergo procedures which put them at risk of acquiring an infection although they do not have an infection at the time of the procedure.

Protozoon: a single-celled micro-organism, usually bigger than a bacterium, which may be free-living or parasitic. Malaria is caused by a protozoon.

Pseudomonas: a bacterium causing a wide variety of infections but most commonly associated with patients whose immunity is impaired by either disease, treatment or indwelling medical equipment and devices.

Salmonella: a bacterium most commonly associated with diarrhoea and food poisoning. There are numerous species, one of which causes typhoid fever.

Staphylococcus: a group of bacteria which cause a wide variety of infections especially of skin and wounds. More serious infections include blood-poisoning and pneumonia as well as heart valve, bone and joint infections.

Streptococcus: a group of bacteria which cause a wide variety of infections including those of skin and wounds. More serious infections include scarlet fever and pneumonia.

Systemic treatment: drugs given by mouth (oral) or injection.

Topical treatment: drugs applied directly, or locally, to the part being treated, for example to the skin or eye.

Treponema pallidum: causative organism of syphilis.

Tuberculosis (TB): an infectious disease most commonly affecting the lungs. Treatment with antibiotics takes many months.

Vaccine: a preparation used to stimulate the development of antibodies and thus confer immunity against a specific disease or diseases.

Virus: a very small micro-organism of simple structure, only capable of survival within a living host cell.

Zoonosis: an infectious disease of animals which can be transmitted to humans.

This glossary is based largely on information supplied by the Association of Medical Microbiologists.

APPENDIX 9

Acronyms

ABPI	Association of the British Pharmaceutical Industry
ACNFP	UK Advisory Committee on Novel Foods and Processes
AIDS	Acquired immune-deficiency syndrome
AMM	UK Association of Medical Microbiologists
APUA	Alliance for the Prudent Use of Antibiotics
ARM	WHO Antimicrobial Resistance Monitoring programme
BBSRC	UK Biotechnology and Biological Sciences Research Council
BMA	British Medical Association
BPMF	British Poultry Meat Federation
BSAC	British Society for Antimicrobial Chemotherapy
CCDC	Consultant in Communicable Disease Control
CDC	US Centers for Communicable Disease Control and Prevention
CDSC	UK Communicable Disease Surveillance Centre
CVL	UK Central Veterinary Laboratory
DH	UK Department of Health
DOT	Directly-observed therapy
EMC	WHO Division of Emerging and other Communicable Diseases Surveillance and Control
EU	European Union
FAO	Food and Agriculture Organization
FDA	US Food and Drug Administration
FEDESA	Fédération Européenne de la Santé Animale
FSIS	US Food Safety Inspection Service
GMO	Genetically modified organism
GP	General practitioner (family doctor)
HACCP	Hazard Analysis at Critical Control Points
HIV	Human immune-deficiency virus
HMO	Health management organisation
ICARE	Intensive Care Antibiotic Resistance Epidemiology
ICNA	UK Infection Control Nurses Association
IT	Information technology
MAFF	UK Ministry of Agriculture, Fisheries and Food
MDR–TB	Multi-drug resistant tuberculosis
MRC	UK Medical Research Council
MRSA	Methicillin-resistant *Staphylococcus aureus*
NCCLS	US National Committee for Clinical Laboratory Standards
NHS	UK National Health Service
NIAID	US National Institute of Allergy and Infectious Diseases
NIBSC	UK National Institute for Biological Standards and Control
NIH	US National Institutes of Health
NOAH	UK National Office of Animal Health Ltd
NNIS	US National Nosocomial Infections Surveillance
OST	UK Office of Science and Technology
OSTP	US Office of Science and Technology Policy
OTC	Over the counter
PhRMA	Pharmaceutical Research and Manufacturers of America
PHLS	UK Public Health Laboratory Service
POM	Prescription-only medicine
POST	Parliamentary Office of Science and Technology
PPA	UK Prescription Pricing Authority
ppm	Parts per million
PRP	Penicillin-resistant *Streptococcus pneumoniae*
RCGP	Royal College of General Practitioners
SKB	SmithKline Beecham
TB	Tuberculosis
UKASTA	UK Agricultural Supply Trade Association

VISA	Vancomycin intermediate-resistant *Staphylococcus aureus*
VLA	UK Veterinary Laboratories Agency
VMD	UK Veterinary Medicines Directorate
VRE	Vancomycin-resistant enterococcus
VRSA	Vancomycin-resistant *Staphylococcus aureus*
WHO	World Health Organization

ISBN 0-10-478998-0

9 780104 789988

Printed in the United Kingdom for The Stationery Office Limited
Dd 5068931 6/99 56219 Job No. J86112